Herbal Antibiotics

Safe Plant Based Herbal Remedies for Fending Off Viral

(Little-known Ways Beginners Can Use Herbalism and Herbal Medicine for Healing)

Monica Wright

Published By **Chris David**

Monica Wright

Herbal Antibiotics: Safe Plant Based Herbal Remedies for Fending Off Viral (Little-known Ways Beginners Can Use Herbalism and Herbal Medicine for Healing)

ISBN 978-1-998901-50-0

Legal & Disclaimer

The information contained in this ebook is not designed to replace or take the place of any form of medicine or professional medical advice. The information in this ebook has been provided for educational & entertainment purposes only.

The information contained in this book has been compiled from sources deemed reliable, and it is accurate to the best of the Author's knowledge; however, the Author cannot guarantee its accuracy and validity and cannot be held liable for any errors or omissions. Changes are periodically made to this book. You must consult your doctor or get professional medical advice before using any of the suggested remedies, techniques, or information in this book.

Upon using the information contained in this book, you agree to hold harmless the Author from and against any damages, costs, and expenses, including any legal fees potentially resulting from the application of any of the information provided by this guide. This disclaimer applies to any damages or injury caused by the use and application, whether directly or indirectly, of any advice or information presented, whether for breach of contract, tort, negligence, personal injury, criminal intent, or under any other cause of action.

You agree to accept all risks of using the information presented inside this book. You need to consult a professional medical practitioner in order to ensure you are both able and healthy enough to participate in this program.

Table Of Contents

Chapter 1: Why Synthetic Antibiotics Are A Big Problem In Today's Society 1

Chapter 2: Often Found In Your Kitchen .. 8

Chapter 3: Herbs.................................... 14

Chapter 4: Extracts................................ 31

Chapter 5: From Plants 39

Chapter 6: From Trees 45

Chapter 7: Best Herbal Choices For Various Ailments.. 48

Chapter 8: Talking With Your Doctor Concerning Herbal Antibiotics................ 52

Chapter 9: Tips For Getting The Best Possible Herbal Antibiotics.................... 54

Chapter 10: Antibiotics 60

Chapter 11: The Immune System........... 93

Chapter 12: Why Healing Naturally...... 123

Chapter 13: Boost Your Immune System With Herbal Medicine 168

Chapter 14: Garlic - A Powerful Antibiotic 170
Chapter 15: Natural Cleaner For Everyday Use.. 181

Chapter 1: Why Synthetic Antibiotics are a Big Problem in Today's Society

In addition, synthetic antibiotics cause severe side consequences, but they also contribute to many issues within our current society. They have actually been viewed as one of the major issues that both science and medicine must take a closer take a look at.

Lack of Information

The main issue is that most people are unaware that there are herbal, natural antibiotics available to them. They think that their doctor knows best, based on the way we've been promoting in the society. If your doctor tells you that you require antibiotics, go to the pharmacy and purchase the antibiotics without asking questions.

For many who read this book, it could be a shocking revelation. Perhaps you're even unhappy that you've spent thousands of dollars on prescription antibiotics, when you could have had alternatives that were less expensive and healthier. You may not have known up until now that they existed or can help you feel better.

Unfortunately, until the society in general is aware about the benefits of natural herbs as an option alternative, the usage of antibiotics made from synthetic will continue to remain.

Liver

The liver is an vital organ of the body. It must function properly to allow us to enjoy our fullest potential. Utilizing synthetic antibiotics frequently can cause damage to the liver. This could make it more difficult for your body to carry out the functions which keep you healthy and in good health.

Interact with Other Medicines

If you're suffering from another health issue it is possible that you are taking prescription medicines. It's possible that they won't work in conjunction with the synthetic antibacterial drugs. You could experience more adverse negative effects, or other medicines may not function equally. This can put you at risk to your overall health.

Dehydration

One of the frequent adverse effect of antibiotics that are synthetic is diarrhea. In the process, dehydration can happen when the body's losing electrolytes and fluids. One may not feel thirsty, however this does not mean that they are hydrated. This is why particular care must be taken.

Vaginal Yeast Infections

Research has linked the increase the incidence of yeast-related vaginal infections with using synthetic antibacterial agents. This is due to the fact that they eliminate good bacteria and bad bacteria. The body is dependent on beneficial bacteria to keep things in balance. Even little girls can suffer from vaginal yeast infections as a reason.

In reality, the way doctors are treating them is to prescribe another antibiotic. This could lead to a cycle that's both painful and harmful. The yeast infection in the vagina can trigger burning, itching and pain.

Creation of Superbugs Due to Resistance

There are medical experts who are concerned that synthetic antibiotics have created superbugs. They make it more difficult and more difficult to effectively manage bacterial infections of a basic nature. The reason is because the body's immune system will begin to develop an immunity to antibiotics. It becomes more difficult to eradicate the disease with the same antibiotics.

This is a particular issue especially for children in the early years, who are more likely to fall ill more often and with greater frequency than adults. If they are treated with synthetic antibiotics frequently but they do not become efficient. This could lead to the simplest bacterial infection becoming into something that needs hospitalization.

Hypersensitivity and Allergies

Some people are not comfortable with taking synthetic antibiotics. The body may develop hypersensitivity or an allergy to an ingredient contained in the drug. For instance, many people are sensitive to penicillin however, they don't realize it until they try it the very first time.

Their faces may become swollen and they might breakout in an rash, or they might experience breathing difficulties. These issues require medical attention and , often, an additional medication to relieve of the signs.

Cost

The price of antibiotics made from synthetic substances is increasing continuously. Even those who have insurance for health are often disappointed with deductibles and co-pays. They may also discover that, when they go into the pharmacy their insurance won't cover the specific antibiotic prescribed.

For instance, amoxicillin is typically covered. But many patients are intolerant to its positive effects because of their body's tolerance to antibiotics. This is why they're given Z-Pac however, it is not often included in health insurance plans.

Risk to Children/Pets

If you use artificial antibiotics at home you pose an opportunity for children as well as pets. There is a risk that they'll come across and consume the antibiotics. A high dose of these medications can be very dangerous and not just for children, but adults too.

Doing more than the suggested dosage will not aid in getting better faster. It is also necessary to adhere to the duration given, even if are feeling better. If you don't, there's possibility that the bacteria will not be eradicated completely and you'll have to begin again with the treatment.

Huge Profits for Companies

The enormous profits pharmaceutical companies earn from sales of synthetic antibiotics adds up in the billions per year.

This is the main reason there isn't any push to encourage consumers to seek out natural antibiotics. These companies prefer to earn money rather than focusing on the overall health of the society.

Chapter 2: Often Found in Your Kitchen

A number of natural herbs that you can select are present in the kitchen. If you or family members suffer from frequently sick with bacterial infections, you can add them to your meals you prepare. They can enhance the flavor of your food and beverages and provide you with an easy way to stay healthy.

Apple Cider Vinegar

There are significant levels of malic acid and acetic acid in the apple cider vinegar. Also, it contains a lot of vitamins and amino acids. It's a great method to combat illness since it is antiviral an antibacterial and anti-fungal.

A spoonful of it each morning and at evening is a fantastic method to combat health issues. If you aren't a fan of the flavor, mix it in water to make it less sour.

Cabbage

The curative properties of cabbage are vast, but the majority of people do not eat it. Include it in your diet at least once per each week for a boost to your immunity. You can also drink freshly squeezed green juice every week to help recover from an problem that has drained your energy.

Coconut Oil

Coconut oil can not only aid in reducing the chance of getting bacteria It also makes the food you cook healthier. It has a variety of health benefits, and also tastes delicious! Every recipe that requires the use of vegetable oil could be healthier by making this easy change. It is possible to use this multiple times per week as a part of a healthy diet. Small adjustments like this that make a difference the most.

Coconut oil can improve the immune system. It also has anti-fungal properties and a wealth of antioxidants. It's believed that it can help increase blood sugar levels and improve the brain's functioning. If you're not looking to prepare meals with it try adding one teaspoon to your cup of coffee each morning to get an energy boost and energy.

Fermented Foods

What is the first thing that comes to mind when you think of fermented food? Most people associate it with alcohol. There are however advantages to eating fermented food because they're classified as probiotics. They destroy harmful bacteria, but not the healthy bacteria in your body.

A few great options within this category of food include pickles that are cultured and raw. It is also possible to take daily capsules of it in your local health food shop. Fermented foods are full of antioxidants as well as necessary microorganisms. They provide greater benefits than capsules.

Garlic

Since the beginning of time, garlic has been utilized all over the globe to treat ailments. It has been utilized to treat throat infections, flu and even for in the case of the Black Plague. Garlic is a potent antioxidant that can destroy harmful bacteria.

It also removes free radicals from the bloodstream and the immune system gets stronger. Allicin is the main ingredient in garlic and it assists in destroying bacteria and viruses, something the prescription antibiotics aren't effective at.

Garlic is a popular ingredient in food as cloves. It is also possible to make into juice. If you do not like the flavor of garlic it is possible to take capsules. You'll only need a small amount to enjoy the benefits, but too excessive garlic could cause stomach upset. If you take any kind of blood thinner medication do not use the garlic in your remedy.

Ginger

Ginger is not just powerful, it also has an extremely strong scent. The aroma is the result of different essential oils and compounds it's composed of. Some of these ingredients have the properties of antibacterial, and antiinflammatory. A small amount of ginger is recommended at one period of.

Honey

The delicious, sweet taste of honey is an item that is a favorite in any kitchen. It also has antibacterial properties. There were many cultures that relied on raw honey prior to the time that the introduction of synthetic antibiotics.

A antimicrobial enzyme can be found in honey. It stops various harmful bacteria from developing. It's also believed to aid in the maintenance of the liver, and reduce the amount of toxins that could harm your immune system. It can also be added into drinks eaten on toast, sprinkled over hot cereals, or eaten as a raw drink.

Onion

Many cook with onion because of its flavor However, they're also helping to boost their immune system. Onion can assist to treat almost everything you can think of. It is believed to help with bacterial infection, and even inflammation.

Onion is a source of sulfur compounds which is why it a great natural antibiotic. They can also help to reduce the symptoms of the common cold and the flu, which are viral--not bacterial--illnesses.

Sage

If you suffer from respiratory infections of the upper part of your body Sage is an excellent solution to make you get more comfortable. Incorporating this into your diet often can strengthen your immunity and guard against health issues that are developing. It doesn't require any sage to make an impact.

Chapter 3: Herbs

There are many herbs that you can use in cooking or for making drinks with herbs. There's a huge list of herbs that provide the benefit from natural anti-microbials. You might already be using one or two of them.

Other herbs you can purchase on the street, either freshly grown or dried. It is essential to try to locate high-quality herbal products. The higher the quality and the stronger they are, the more can provide in fighting off infections caused by bacteria.

Allspice

It is a potent antioxidant and anti-inflammatory components Allspice is definitely a factor to think about when it comes to herbal antibiotics. It is a great ingredient to use in many recipes, and is frequently a preventive aid. It may give the immune system a boost , so you're less likely get bacterial infections as well as other illnesses. It's extremely potent. only a small amount is a significant amount of the flavor.

Anise

This spice is typically employed in Asian cuisine, but it can be used in any dish. It's not necessary to use a lot of it, it has strong taste. It is similar to licorice and it's often confused with the former in food items.

Anise has been utilized as a remedy for healing for centuries throughout Asia and throughout the globe. Its antibacterial properties are only one of the benefits it can provide. It also contains a lot of antioxidants.

Do not exceed 500 mg daily. If you plan to take the maximum dosage split it into three or two doses over the day, rather than all at one time.

Basil

Incorporate basil into most of the food you cook to increase your immunity. Basil oil can be added to food items you don't cook, like salads. It can help you keep your health in check and, should you ever suffer from a bacteria-related infection, it will aid in eliminating harmful bacteria in the early stages of.

Bay Leaf

The many benefits of bay leaf makes it a preferred choice for people fighting infections caused by bacteria. It also aids in reducing stomach issues and acne. The oil of bay leaves aids in reducing the capacity for harmful bacteria multiply. It also helps fight the development of various kinds of fungi.

Cardamom

One of the most secrets to combating harmful bacteria is the use of cardamom. It's a great source of cineol. It's also a popular method to combat persistent bad breath.

This is an extremely beneficial herb to treat coughing and sore throat. It is not recommended to use cardamom when you suffer from gallstones or when your gall bladder is removed.

Caraway Seed

The best results when you search for caraway seeds that are black. Since the beginning of time it has been used to aid in a wide range of health problems. It's a great way to combat the bacterial causes of deep infections that are difficult to treat.

The oil is best taken at the time you experience the first symptoms of health issues. You can take a teaspoon of it in the morning and another at night , until the symptoms have disappeared. If you do not like the flavor then add a teaspoon of honey in the mix. The recommended daily dosage for prevention is 50 to 100 mg.

Chervil

Chervil's history runs deeply in various different cultures throughout the world. It is a wild plant that grows in numerous areas and it took only a few years for its value to be recognized. The most effective method to utilize it is to boil a few leaves of chervil in a glass of vinegar made from apple cider. Take the leaves off and then drink the concoction along with a couple of spoons of honey to sweeten it.

Chervil is a good option for people suffering from chronic cough. This type of cough makes it difficult to fall asleep at the end of the night. Drinking a cup of tea of this herb prior to attempting to fall asleep can help you get the sleep you require.

Chili Peppers

There are a variety of kinds of chili peppers there for you to choose from. Some have mild heat, while others possess moderate or very hot heat. There is no need to consume a lot of these peppers to benefit from the benefits. They can help keep your body healthy and prevent harmful bacteria from forming.

Cinnamon

To sweeten things, you can find cinnamon, which can also provide protection from harmful bacteria. Cinnamon can be utilized in the baking of various sweets or sprinkled into drinks to enhance their sweetness without sugar. It may help to reduce the symptoms of common cold and muscle spasms, vomiting and inflammation.

Cloves

In addition to helping fight infections caused by bacteria, they also help to alleviate the pain. By placing a few cloves cooked inside your mouth between the gums and teeth can decrease inflammation and pain until you are seen at the dentist.

Cloves are also used to alleviate mild pain from inflammation, like arthritis-related symptoms. Cloves can aid in reducing nausea and vomiting caused by illnesses like the flu, health issues and even the side consequences of prescription drugs.

Coriander

One of the most well-known uses of coriander is that it can reduce the chance from food poisoning. It is also a great aid in fighting different kinds of infections which appear to be intolerant to antibiotics prescribed by doctors. (This resistance may occur when people take antibiotics too often). You can mix it into nearly every food item and it will not alter the flavor.

Joint pain is usually decreased by using coriander. Many people have found that it naturally helps to treat hemorrhoids. Women who are nursing or pregnant could use it to boost the flow of milk.

Cumin

The addition of a tiny amount of cumin in your food can enhance the flavor. This is particularly true for Peruvian cuisines. Cumin is an effective anti-microbial option. It is a source of thymol which can help improve the effectiveness prescribed antibiotics if you are required to take them.

Dill

A small amount of dill will go far because of the tangy taste it imparts to food items. Dill also helps your body fight illnesses and improve your immunity. Dill is available fresh in the summer months and during the during the first part of autumn. You can also find dried dill throughout the year. Dill can also be beneficial in fighting bone loss.

It is a good idea to apply it on the inside of the throat or mouth to ease discomfort. It is essential not to apply dill if the medication you take is lithium according to what the doctor has advised. Dill could result in your system not making lithium as it is supposed to.

Fennel

A lot of people add fennel seeds into their meals or on salads to boost their metabolism. It is a popular ingredient for long-lasting weight loss. Fennel also has anti-fungal as well as antibacterial properties.

Lemon Balm

Lemon balm does not only smell and taste delicious, it's also antibacterial. It also is a relaxing herbal remedy that's been extensively used to ease anxiety and stress. It is available as a tea dried leaves, capsules and extracts. Lemon balm should not be taken by those who take thyroid medication.

Marjoram

Common colds can prove debilitating however, marjoram is a great option to decrease the amount of time it lasts. It helps with both viral and bacterial illnesses. It is so gentle that many parents utilize it with their infants and children. It is also efficient enough to provide assistance for adultstoo. It's available as an oil along with dried leaves.

Marjoram is typically used in teas which can be offered to children to help ease the symptoms of the symptoms of a runny nose, or symptoms of common cold. It is also utilized to treat dry coughs that appear to last for a long time. Sore throat and ear pain throat are additional reasons to take marjoram.

Mints

Mints contain a variety of essential oils that help to boost the immune system as well as soothe the digestive tract. They can be utilized in the various foods you purchase at the supermarket in order to increase the shelf life. Mints can be used in conjunction with tea, in form of leaves or oil to reduce the risk of the risk of bacterial infections. This includes infections which affect the throat and the sinuses.

Mustard

Mustard seeds can be used in many delicious food items. Only a small amount to enjoy the benefits they bring. Even the mild mustard condiment has these seeds, and it has antibacterial qualities to provide.

Use of mustard could assist in relieving the inflammation and pain in muscles. It's also a great alternative to treat the common cold. The leaves of black mustard are utilized in salads as well as other food items. Also, you can use capsules to reap the benefits, or cook mustard seeds for tea.

Nutmeg

There are numerous ways to use Nutmeg, in addition to giving flavor to food items. Many people use it in desserts and sweets It can also be added to any type of food items. It is often utilized to combat E. Staph and E. coli infections. It is a natural antimicrobial that can assist in the reduction of harmful bacteria.

Nutmeg is also a great remedy for mouth sores and joint pain. It can also help with diarrhea and nausea. Limit your use to 120 mg per day , or it could cause hallucinations.

Oregano

Oregano isn't just used to enhance the flavor of your favourite Italian dishes. It also helps to keep your health in check due to its antibacterial properties that it offers. The oil extracted from the leaves of oregano is the one with the greatest potential.

It's been compared to what penicillin can offer by way of prescription antibiotic penicillin. Certain studies have shown that oregano is able to kill prostate cancerous cells. Oregano's use can be extremely beneficial for respiratory tract problems such as cough, croup, and asthma.

In the case of such conditions for such conditions, the recommended dose is 200 mg daily. This should not be taken by people who are taking medications to treat bleeding disorders.

Parsley

There are some proven anti-bacterial properties that can be observed in parsley. It is primarily derived from the oil that is extracted from the parsley seeds. It is able to fight various kinds of fungi and bacteria. One of the ailments that parsley can treat is staph infections.

It is also utilized to treat and prevent UTIs (UTIs) and also to ease the discomfort caused by kidney stones. It may reduce the length of time that a common cold persists, and also reduce the chance of developing jaundice. It is commonly used to treat children who suffer from colic.

Pepper

There are many varieties of pepper you can make use of to reduce the possibility of bacteria, or to combat them. This includes chili pepper, black pepper, and cayenne. They also aid in combating intestinal issues and.

All peppers contain capsicum and it is this that combats the bacteria. The more hot the pepper the stronger it will be at fighting off the bacteria. However, it is important to ensure that the food items you add pepper to do not become too hot to consume.

Rosemary

One essential oil which smells wonderful is rosemary. It can be applied to treat the body or inhaled via an infuser. If you decide to use an essential oils, then you will only require a few drops since they're extremely potent. Do not add more than 2 drops of it in your bathwater.

Rosemary has amazing effects on your immune system. It is a kind of aromatherapy which can be utilized to treat chronic asthma-related issues. It is able to fight bacteria, mold and fungi.

Sage

Reduced inflammation and stopping the spread of the effects of bacterial infections are among the most well-known advantages of Sage. It is generally sold in dried form that is cooked. But, the leaves could be also boiled and strain to create a robust tea.

There are some experts who believe that daily consumption of sage may help reduce the risk of developing Alzheimer's disease and diabetes. It's often utilized to ease the discomfort and pressure caused by an infection of the sinuses. It is a great way to lessen the dry cough as well as swelling in the airways due to asthma , bronchitis or other respiratory conditions. The dose should not exceed 2.5 mg.

Tarragon

In the beginning, tarragon was considered an anti-biotic that was naturally produced to stop food poisoning from occurring in various meals. It was regarded as a superior preserver that let food be stored longer without causing illness to consumers. Tarragon was also an early treatment for intestinal problems as well as to fight tuberculosis.

It is also an easy way to help promote healthier sleeping habits. A lot of people feels tired and sluggish when they use over-the-counter and prescription sleeping aids. Tarragon will help you rest comfortably without having that side effect that you have to manage.

The dosage to be taken will depend on the age of the person and degree of the illness. It is suggested to begin with an amount of medication and then check how it performs for you. Increase the dosage gradually as needed for the greatest advantages.

Thyme

Another method of cooking and helping to reduce bacterial issues is the herb thyme. It is commonly used to treat persistent dry coughing. It is also a valuable source for people suffering from breathing disorders, including asthma or bronchitis. The herb can aid in soothing the digestive tract, too.

Thyme is a great remedy for whooping cough, even if it's affecting children. It can help treat laryngitis and sore throat. If the tonsils are swelling and painful, it may help in decreasing inflammation and pain.

Turmeric

A common spice present in food items that originate from across the Middle East is turmeric. The primary ingredients provide the capability to block enzymes that enable harmful bacteria to multiply. Turmeric contains properties that to reduce inflammation, bacterial infections and other forms of chronic diseases. It also helps with chronic headaches and bronchitis.

Although turmeric can be hot, it could be an effective natural remedy for heartburn. For those who like spicy food but don't want suffering from the effects, this could be the perfect solution! It also helps decrease inflammation and pain moderate to mild arthritis.

Chapter 4: Extracts

You may have heard of the advantages of various extracts. They typically come in capsules that have ingredients designed to enhance your overall well-being and health. If you are already taking some of these extracts daily as an supplement, you're fighting off infections caused by bacteria without ever realizing that you are doing it!

They're not expensive and can result in an enormous difference in how you feel. Think about the benefits these extracts can provide to you so that you can choose the one that's best suited to your requirements.

Colloidal Silver

The many properties of colloidal silver are aimed at killing germs and bacteria. The supplement, that is an element is utilized for over 100 years to kill fungi and bacteria. It is also used to treat various viruses.

Silver colloidal can also aid in the healing process of open sores and wounds that aren't healing in the way they ought to. It is extremely beneficial for people who suffer from asthma. It may also boost energy for those who are suffering from chronic fatigue.

Minerals like this is best used in very small quantities. Follow the directions for use provided on the package of the supplement. The strength of colloidal silver may differ from one supplement to the next.

Chrysanthemum Lavandulifolium Extract

This extract is very identical structure to synthetic antibiotics. The theory is that it was among the oldest medicines that have been used in different cultures to treat ailments. It is also able to strengthen the immune system through encouraging the growth of healthy cells.

Echinacea

The time it takes to heal of a bacterial infection or fungal infection could be cut down by the use of the echinacea. It is a great aid in reducing the duration and symptoms of respiratory infections, ear sinus infections, and other sinus issues. It also decreases inflammation, which means that it will not be as severe.

A majority of people use echinacea as a capsule-based supplement. If the oil is taken in a small amount, it should be taken by putting a teaspoon into one glass of water every day. Many people make echinacea tea using the addition of a little honey to enhance the flavor.

Grapefruit Seed Extract

The potent antioxidants that are found in grapefruit are well-known. But there are many who aren't an avid fan of the fruit in its fresh form or juice. Some prefer to sweeten the juice with lots of sugar, which can lead to health issues later on.

An effective solution is intake of grapefruit seed extract. It is a source of anti-fungal and antibacterial properties. The results of studies have revealed more than 800 varieties of bacteria as well as over 100 kinds of bacteria that can be destroyed with this supplement. The best part, however is that it will not harm the healthy bacteria that your body requires.

Lavender Oil

A lot of people depend on lavender oil to help rest and sleep better. It is popular for its ability to reduce inflammation. It also has antibacterial extract that helps to treat sinus infections, respiratory issues and bacterial infections which affect the throat and ears.

Lavender oil has the ability to reduce the severity of inflammation throughout the body, both in terms of intensity and duration. It is only a matter of the smallest amount of lavender oil since it's very powerful. It is possible to add drops of lavender oil to bath water or add them to diffusers.

Neem Oil

A tiny quantity of the neem oil will go far in bringing health benefits. The oil is derived from the neem plant. It is also possible for purchase, however this oil has the greatest beneficial effects for your body. Neem has been utilized for over 4000 centuries across India as well as Africa to improve skin conditions and cut down on the time it takes for your body's healing process.

Neem oil is also able to slow the growth of bacteria and viruses. In addition it's a natural pain reliever , and it helps to decrease inflammation. It is able to reduce the fever of a person within a short time. Most often, it is employed to decrease the symptoms of nausea and upset stomachs, which could be the an adverse effect of a variety of prescribed medications.

Pau d'Arco

A lot of people think that pau d'arco originates from France because of its name, however it actually comes from South America. The primary ingredient in this plant is lapachol. It can help reduce the effects of infections caused by fungus, bacteria and viruses. Many experts believe that it contains properties that could assist in the fight against certain forms of cancer.

But, the majority of people are using it to treat common cold symptoms. There are some who claim that when they take pau d'arco right away when they begin to feel the first signs of a cold, they'll be in good shape within a few days. They don't feel the acuity of the cold and it doesn't last for long.

Some people opt to take the low dose of pau di'arco in the flu and cold season. They do this as an opportunity to improve the immune system, and lower the likelihood of contracting illness. This is particularly true for people who work with a lot of people, since they are more vulnerable to the illnesses that are transmitted by air.

Seed Nut Extract

Although extracts of nut seeds are frequently used to manage the effects of diabetes, this extract also contains lots of antioxidants. It is a great way to combat problems related to glycemic index (GI) or chronic infections caused by bacteria.

It is possible to buy seed nuts in capsule form to be taken regularly as a form of prevention. The most beneficial benefits are from the oil taken from the seeds of the nuts. The essential oil is potent and therefore you will only require the drops of it at one time.

Tea Tree Oil

The oil of tea tree was utilized by doctors and medical professionals up until the 1940s , when they began using penicillin. However, it is considered to be to be one of the top natural antibiotics on the market. It is derived from the leaves of the plant, which originated in New South Wales and Australia. It is antibacterial as well as antiviral. It has enough potency to combat MRSA and other infections of staff.

The essential oil is powerful and must be used with caution. A drop or two is needed to achieve results. The leaves can be used to boil the leaves, however the most effective results are obtained from the oil extracted version.

Chapter 5: From Plants

A variety of natural antibiotics are derived from plants. They were employed by people of the past to stop illnesses and treat various diseases. They also can help to maintain your health or combat a an infection caused by bacteria.

Aloe Vera

The aloe vera is among the plants that people use to soothe burns. This includes cooking burns as well as sunburns. The plant thrives in climates which are dry and hot. It also helps fight infections caused by bacteria and herpes.

For aloe use, cut the leaves off of the plant and extract the sap out of it. You can then boil it and inhale the vapors that help your body recover from illnesses. To treat burns, it's placed directly on the burn region. A few people make Aloe Juice and consume it in order to increase their immunity.

There are also capsules made of aloe to treat an various health issues. The recommended daily dose is between 100 to 200 mg daily.

Cryptolepis

It is a flowering plant found in Gambia as well as Congo. Cryptolepis is extracted from the roots and leaves. It is commonly utilized for treating the symptoms of type II diabetes and malaria. The antibacterial components make it an extremely potent weapon to fight infections and harmful bacteria.

Cryptolepis is available in various forms. The capsules and powder are the most popular. The tea is beneficial to the body however the flavor can be bitter. The addition of nectar or honey may enhance the flavor.

Echinacea

Since the beginning of time, echinacea has been used to provide the immune system with some support. It's also been employed to combat infections that are of the viral and bacterial varieties. It's a powerful herb, and it has the ability to eliminate serious strains of bacteria, like those that cause staph and MRSA.

Echinacea appears to be one of the most popular natural antibiotics that are a go-to. It is due to its ability to help with a variety of health issues. It is a good idea to take it regularly in small doses to combat viral and bacterial infections. It is also a good option to reach promptly if you notice that you are experiencing an illness.

Many people report that echinacea can help them feel more relaxed. There aren't many people who don't experience an improvement in their health when using it. There are capsules and liquid versions available at the majority of grocery stores that sell health foods.

Eucalyptus

The oil produced by Eucalyptus has been used throughout the globe for hundreds of years. It is indigenous to Australia and is used for its antiseptic properties in pharmaceuticals. For extraction of the oil the leaves are either boiled or steam.

The extraction process is lengthy and laborious. This is the reason it's costly. Eucalyptus oils should not be applied directly on the skin, without diluting. If you do this it may cause burning and itching on the skin. The negative side effects could outweigh the positive effects, so be sure to dilute the oil. The oil should not be taken orally.

This is a fantastic alternative for people who haven't experienced success with other antibiotics from herbal sources or any improvement from the synthetic ones. These health issues can be chronic sinus infections, as well as ear infections.

Juniper

The juniper plant has become recognized for the delicious fruits it produces. They can be found in a variety of drinks and foods to provide flavor. It's an antibiotic version of herbal medicine that is frequently neglected. It is a great way to reduce the problems related to inflammation or bronchitis. It also helps fight bacteria that cause infections.

To benefit your health it is a great option. The dosage is approximately 100 mg daily. If you're using actual fruit, the dose is only 1 g per day. It can be difficult to find fresh Juniper berries year-round However, oil can be purchased on the internet or at an organic store.

Licorice

The delicious smell and flavor of licorice make it appealing for both adults and children. It has antibacterial and anti-fungal properties. It is commonly utilized to treat inflammation. It is an excellent option for chronic viral and bronchitis.

Licorice can boost in strengthening the immune system, so it is a great remedy to combat common colds and flu. It's best to take tiny amounts however. The whole root is the most potent medicinal benefits. It should not be used by those suffering from high blood pressure.

If you suffer from trouble with your throat, or have strep throat then making tea with honey and licorice root could help soothe the pain quickly. Mix 1 tablespoon of the licorice root powder for 8 eight ounces of boiling water. Drink two times a day until you feel better.

Olive Leaf

It is not difficult to see the many benefits that come from olive leaf. They include reducing inflammation and removing harmful bacteria and improving immunity. It is frequently employed by those suffering from digestive issues and arthritis.

The recommended daily dose for treating ongoing health issues is 30 milliliters. For prevention, the dosage ranges from 10 to 20 milliliters per day. It can be administered by mouth in liquid form, however it is not recommended to exceed 2 tablespoons daily.

Chapter 6: From Trees

There are a few natural antibiotics are derived from trees. Although this list is a bit more limited and less popular however, that doesn't mean it makes these options less accessible or unavailable.

Goldenseal Root

Although goldenseal root isn't popular as other natural antibiotics, it should not be ignored. It's a great option to win against bacteria and fungus. It also helps decrease chronic inflammation. This is a powerful plant that can help reduce throat swelling rapidly.

It helps to soothe the lining of mucous membranes that may become inflamed due to respiratory issues or sinus infections. Goldenseal root may also help to ease the dry cough that can interfere with sleep.

Poke Root

The Poke root appears very bizarre and grows in the fertile soil regions that are found in North America. It is beneficial in fighting off bacteria and helping the immune system get some assistance. It is important to be cautious when making use of it however, because the excessive amount of poke root may cause poisoning. Limit yourself to one drop per day , or it could cause kidney damage.

Usnea

Most commonly referred to as an antioxidant, usnea can also be an excellent way to fight harmful bacteria. It also helps keep different types of fungus in check and maintain an excellent immune system. This is an excellent alternative for those suffering from an ongoing cough. Usnea reduces mucus membranes.

Woodworm

Woodworm is mostly used to treat infections caused by worms, it is also used to aid in treating Crohn's disease and inflammation issues. It is an herb-based anti-inflammatory that aids the body fight viral and bacterial infections.

It is an oil that's essential and should be taken in small doses. It can be purchased in capsules as well. Limit yourself to 5 grams of this ingredient daily.

Chapter 7: Best Herbal Choices for Various Ailments

Finding the most effective herbal anti-biotics to treat various ailments is essential. Although most have the ability to eliminate harmful bacteria, some help to fight harmful fungus and viruses. They also improve your immune system.

Every person reacts to herbal antibiotics in a different way. This is due to the fact that each person's body's chemistry is unique. It is possible to play with a couple of different alternatives before you discover what works best for you to stay good health or as preventative.

What you decide to use can also be different according to the health conditions that you're dealing with. If you aren't feeling well, you require an immediate solution that will help you feel at you're at your optimal in the shortest period of time.

To successfully combat infections caused by viruses and bacteria it is essential to do everything you can to feel at your most at your best. It is important to understand the advantages of herbal solutions. Here's a brief checklist of resources that you'll discover useful.

Acne: aloe vera, calendula and tea tree oil

* Alcohol use -- kudzu, primrose

* Allergies -Chamomile

* Alzheimer's disease Ginkgo bilbao and rosemary

* Angina -hawthorn, garlic green tea and willow

* Anxiety -- chamomile hops Kava, lavender, passion flower and valerian

* Arthritis capsicum, turmeric, ginger

* Athlete's Foot tea oil from trees

* Bronchitis -- echinacea

* Burns -- aloe vera

* Common cold andrographis and echinacea root

* Cough Eucalyptus

* Depression St. John's wort

* Diarrhea -- bilberry, raspberry

* Dizziness gingko, ginger

* Earache -- echinacea

* Eczema -- chamomile

* Flu -- echinacea

* Gingivitis -Green tea, goldenseal

* Hay fever butter bur

* Blood pressure that is highhawthorn, garlic

* Apples with high cholesterol cinnamon, flaxseed, and apple

* Hot flashes - soy, red clover

* Indigestion -- chamomile, ginger, peppermint

* Infection -- echinacea, garlic, ginseng, tea tree oil

* Hops, insomnia, valerian, kava

* Lower back paincaracole, thymol willow bark

"Migraines" -- Butterbur feverfew

* Morning sickness -- ginger

* Muscle pain capsicum and wintergreen

* Nausea -- ginger

* Sore throat Mullein, licorice

* Stuffy nose -- echinacea

* Toothache -- oil of clove willow

* Yeast infection -- garlic, goldenseal, pau d'arco

Chapter 8: Talking with your Doctor Concerning Herbal Antibiotics

Don't be afraid if you want to speak with your physician about natural antibiotics. With the knowledge that you've learned here it is possible to test some remedies in lieu of synthetic antibiotics.

You must have a strong relationship with your doctor so that you can talk to them in a transparent manner. Tell your doctor the reasons you're planning to take a look at the natural antibiotics. Remember that there might be times that you or someone else in your family requires prescription.

You can also inform your physician that you're going to explore natural antibiotics for both prevention as well as treatment. If you're unable to control the bacteria making you sick, go back to the doctor for a check-up and consider the synthetic antibiotics should they be deemed essential.

The majority of doctors are likely to be able to accept your choice. You can include notes in your medical records and those for your children. They will be grateful for your honesty, and will request you to inform them should you have any concerns or worries.

Medical professionals generally support the use of natural antibiotics. But they're not capable of promoting their products to their clients due to the nature of business. If you're seeing a physician who is trying to convince you to not make use of herbal antibiotics, then you might be thinking about reconsidering the choice of whom you go to for medical advice.

Even if they do not agree with your decision, the majority of medical professionals will be willing to accept your decisions. It is essential that you and your physician to be in agreement regarding your health care needs as well as the family's needs. Do not hide the fact that your use natural antibiotics from your physician.

Chapter 9: Tips for Getting the Best Possible Herbal Antibiotics

It is vital to recognize how the grade of herbal antibiotics can affect their value and efficacy. It's sensible to ensure you have the highest quality choices. Don't compromise on quality and result in something that doesn't function as it ought to.

Research Before You Buy

Don't think that one product is exactly the same as every other. Be a knowledgeable consumer. Make sure you do your homework prior to purchasing any herbicides. Make sure to read reviews online to find out what others have to say about the product.

Also, read the ingredients as you can be surprised by what's often added that you do not wish to have. Be attentive to reviews on the internet from actual consumers. They're superior to testimonials on products. Reviews from customers tell you the product they purchased, what they did with the product and the results they got from it.

Although herbal antibiotics perform differently for different people depending on their chemical constitution You can get a sense of what might work for you. If it works well for the majority of applications this is a great product to think about trying.

Credible Online Sites

It is possible to score some incredible bargains on herbal antibiotics if you buy them on the internet. However, you must to buy the antibiotics from a reputable online store.

Find out how long the company has been in operation for. It is important to remember that anyone can build an attractive and professional website. It is important to know the time span they've been operating and the amount of complaints they've received.

Are you provided with an order tracking number when your order is shipped? What is the standard of their customer service? Are there any kind of warranty or refund policies?

Make sure you compare various websites to gain a real-world understanding of the services offered. Be sure to compare the cost of shipping and pricing as well. Sometimes, you'll get an affordable price, but when you add the shipping cost, you will see a significant increase in the overall price.

If you are able to find a way to input a coupon discount or coupon code, open another browser and search for one. By copying and pasting the information you discover, you'll save money every time you purchase.

Buy Fresh Herbs When Possible

If you are planning to make use of the herbs that you can cook with your antibiotics from your herbs Try to purchase them in fresh. You might be able to purchase them from the produce section of your supermarket. It is dependent on the time of the year there might be farmer markets in your area that sell these.

Keep in mind that adding fresh herbs to your meals that you cook is an excellent line of defense against viral and bacterial health problems. The herbs can also enhance the flavor of the meals you prepare for your family.

Grow Your Own Herbs

There are also kits that you can buy to help to grow your own plants. It's less expensive than purchasing them fresh locally. There isn't a huge area to plant these plants. Actually the kits are so small to fit on the window sill inside your home kitchen.

Follow Dosage Instructions Completely

Do not exceed the dosage prescriptions for herbal antibiotics. Many times, people take more medication thinking that they will improve their health faster. It's not true, and can cause adverse effects or even serious illness.

When you have a dosage that has two options: high and low begin with the lowest dosage you can possibly take. If you aren't sure if you're receiving the greatest benefits, you may gradually increase the amount until you are at the right threshold. If the instructions say to divide the product into three or two doses per day, do not do it all at once.

Proper Storage

Be sure to store your herbal antibiotics. Generallyspeaking, you should protect them from light, heat and humidity. Do not store your supplements in your bathroom because of the moisture created when you shower. Do not place any medication or herbal supplements on the counter so that they are subjected to sun.

Instead, keep them in a dark, cool area that is dry. Keep a good eye on expiration dates, too. Keep any herbal supplements as well as other medications out of reach of children or pets.

Using Essential Oils

The effectiveness in essential oil is essential to know. A few drops of essential oils diluted in water could be far more potent than you think. The majority of essential oils should not be applied directly on the face without diluting. They shouldn't be taken orally also.

Don't mix essential oils in the absence of the instructions of a particular recipe. In the event that you mix essential oils, you may cause certain adverse reactions that aren't pleasant and won't help you reach your health objectives.

Chapter 10: Antibiotics

Is there an antibiotic?

Anything that inhibits the replication and development of a bacterium, or that executes it throughout is known as an anti-toxin. Antibiotics are an antimicrobial designed to fight bacteria that cause disease inside (or within) your body. This is why Antibiotics agents not exactly identical to the other types of antimicrobials that are widely used nowadays:

* Antiseptics can be used to clean tissues that are living when the risk of contamination is high such as, for instance, during medical procedures.

Disinfectants are antimicrobials that are not specific to any particular species that kill a variety of living things on a small scale as well as microscopic organisms. They are used on non-living surfaces, such as for example, in hospitals.

It is evident that microscopic organisms aren't by any way the only microorganisms which can cause harm to us. Infections and organisms can also cause harm to individuals and are focused on antivirals and antifungals in isolation. The only substances that target microorganisms are known as Antibiotics agents. The term antimicrobial is a broad word that refers to anything that hinders or kills microbial cells which includes Antibiotics and antifungals, as well as synthetic compounds and antivirals like germ killers.

The majority of Antibiotics products are administered in research facilities however, they are usually based on mixtures that which scientists have observed in the natural world. Certain organisms, like bacteria create substances specifically to perform another microorganisms to gain the position they prefer while searching in search of water, nourishment or other resources that are limited. However, some microorganisms produce Antibiotics substances in laboratories.

How do you accomplish the Antibiotics agent's task?

Antibiotics are used to treat bacterial illnesses. Some are very specific and work only against certain microbes. Others, referred to as broad range Antibiotics are able to attack a broad range of microorganisms, which includes those that are beneficial to us.

There are two main ways that Antibiotics agents are able to target microscopic organisms. They either stop the proliferation of microbes or kill the microbes, for example, by stopping the part responsible for creating cell dividers.

Why are Antibiotics agents important?

The introduction of Antibiotics agents in medicine changed the way that illnesses that are irresistible were treated. In the time between 1945 and 1972, the Natural human progress accelerated by eight years. Antibiotics were utilized to treat diseases that were already susceptible to kill patients. In the present, Antibiotics agents are one of the most well-known kinds of medicines used in medicine and allow many perplexing treatments that've become Natural across the globe.

If we ran out of feasible Antibiotics The current medications could be impacted by years of. Minor medical procedures, like appendectomy, can become dangerous, just similar to how they were prior Antibiotics became generally available. Antibiotics are often used in a small number of patients prior to surgical procedures to ensure that patients do not contract illnesses from microorganisms in the wounds. Without this protection measure and the risk of blood damage would become much more heightened, and a huge variety of the more difficult medical procedures that doctors currently carry out could not be feasible.

Side Effects and Dangers

Stomach upset

A variety of Antibiotics result in stomach steam or other gastrointestinal issues. This can be caused by:

* nausea

* indigestion

* vomiting

* diarrhea

* Bloating

* sensation of completeness

* Loss of appetite

* stomach cramps or pain

Penicillins, Macrolide antimicrobials, and fluoroquinolones can cause stomach upset more than other Antibiotics.

What to do

Consult your primary doctor or specialist in drugs, whether you can supplement your antimicrobial with food. Consuming food can lessen stomach symptoms caused by certain

Antibiotics drugs, like amoxicillin and doxycycline.

However it isn't a good idea for all Antibiotics. Some Antibiotics agents, like antibiotics, have to be consumed with an empty stomach.

Discuss with your physician to be sure that you know what you need to do with your medication, and what other methods to ease stomach discomfort.

When to contact your primary doctor

The bowels are loose and mellow. The problem will go away once you have stopped taking the medicine. However, if the run-like symptoms are extremely severe, it may result in:

* abdominal pain and squeezes

* fever

* nausea

* blood or mucus that is present in your stool

These symptoms can be caused by the abundance of microbes that are not immune in your digestive tracts. In these instances, call your primary physician immediately.

Photosensitivity

If you're taking an anti-toxindrug, such as antibiotics the body could appear to be more sensitive to light. This can cause lighting appear more attractive to your eyes. This could also make your skin more susceptible to be burned by sunlight.

Photosensitivity should be gone once you've finished with the anti-toxin.

What to do

If you are aware that you'll be on the open air, you can make it safe to stay sheltered and comfortable.

Be sure to apply sunscreen that has UVA and UVB security. Reapply sunscreen in accordance with the label.

In addition, you should wear protective attire and other accessories, like glasses and a cap.

Fever

The symptom of fever is a common occurrence of many drugs, such as Antibiotics. The reason for a fever could be because of an adversely vulnerable reaction to a drug or as a symptom that is terribly unpleasant.

Medication fevers can occur regardless of the anti-toxin used, but they're more frequent with the following:

* beta-lactams

* cephalexin

* minocycline

* sulfonamides

What to do

If you develop a fever taking an anti-toxinmedication, it's likely to leave you alone. If your fever persists after up to 48 hours, learn more about the use of medications for torment relief that are available over the counter like Acetaminophen, or ibuprofen to reduce the severity of your fever.

When should you call your PCP?

If you are suffering from a fever that is more significant that 100degF (38degC) or the appearance of a skin rash or difficulty breathing, contact your doctor immediately.

Vaginal yeast infection

Antibiotics reduce the amount of microorganisms that support the body such as lactobacillus inside the vagina. These "great microorganisms" aids in keeping a naturally occurring growth known as Candida hidden. If this Natural equalization process is being tipped to Candida growth it is possible that yeast contamination will occur.

The side effects are:

* vaginal sensation of tingling

* burning while peeing or during sex

* swelling of the vagina

* soreness

* pain during sex

* redness

* Rash

A clumpy, whitish-dim appearance and a clu from the vagina , now and again referred to like curds is another indicator that you might have yeast-related issues.

What to do

For simple yeast infections Your primary doctor might suggest vaginal antifungal cream or salve, tablet, or oral tablet. Examples include:

* butoconazole

* clotrimazole

* miconazole

* terconazole

* fluconazole

A large number of creams, salves, or Supplpositories are available without the need for a remedy.

If you have serious yeast disorders that are confounded Your primary physician might recommend a more prolonged period of prescription therapy.

In the event that the infection recurs the same way, your partner may also be suffering from yeast disease. It is recommended to use condoms when you are having sexual relations in the event that you suspect that both are suffering from yeast.

Communications with doctors

Certain Natural medicines work with certain Antibiotics agents. This includes:

* blood thinners

* birth control medications (may occur with rifamycins)

* antacids

* antihistamines

* multivitamins, and some enhancements, especially ones that are high in zinc iron, calcium, and zinc

* Non-steroidal calming medications (NSAIDs)

* psoriasis drugs

* rheumatoid joint pain drugs

* diuretics

* antifungals

* diabetes drugs

* Relaxants for muscles

* Steroids

* Parkinson's disease drugs

* Cyclosporine

* lithium

* Retinoids and nutritional Enhancements

* cholesterol-lowering drugs, such as statins

* migraine drugs

* Gout medications

* tricyclic antidepressants

People should always notify a doctor or specialist about any medication they are taking in order to keep a safe distance from any connections. The information in the package must also list the medications that can work with the specific type of Antibiotics.

Photosensitivity

There are many types of Antibiotics cause the skin to become more sensitive to sunlight (photosensitive).

When taking Antibiotics which may trigger photosensitivity, patients must:

* Avoid delays in the time of light introduction

Always use high-SPF, broad-spectrum sunscreens whenever you are in the sun.

* dress in protective attire when you are in the sun, like caps, long-sleeved shirts, caps and long jeans

Anyone who has noticed an unusual effects to any of the above when taking Antibiotics must consult a doctor.

Recoloration of bone and teeth

There are a few studies that suggest that between 3 and 6 percent of people who are taking antibiotics create discolorations on their lacquer teeth. The recoloring can't be reversed in adults, due to how their teeth cannot grow back or change.

The coloration can also be seen on specific bones. However the bones are continually recovering themselves, and so the stains on bones caused through Antibiotics agents are often reverseable.

Talk to a dentist regarding exchanging prescriptions when you are Antibiotics substances causes teeth staining or recoloring.

Hypersensitivity

In rare instances, Antibiotics agents can cause an extremely hypersensitive response called hypersensitivity.

Hypersensitivity can be identified by:

* a heartbeat that is fast

* Hives or an irritated, red skin rash

* anxiety-related feelings and an unsettling

* sensations of tingling and instability

Hives, general irritation on large areas of the body

* swelling of the skin

The swelling can be seen in the throat, mouth and the face

* severe wheezingand hacking, and discomfort relaxing

* Low circulatory strain

* fainting

* seizures

Hypersensitivity, in general occurs within 15 minutes after the use of an antimicrobial. However it can last up to an hour, or even more so following a certain amount.

Hypersensitivity could be fatal if not treated with immediate crisis treatment. If people suspect hypersensitivity, they should call the crisis helpline or visit the crisis room right away.

Resistance to antibiotics and addiction

Applying hand sanitizers as if they're going out of fashion (shockingly however, they're not) and then popping Antibiotics drugs at the first sign of illness. Without even knowing the consequences, many people engage in unproductive antibacterial excess.

Although the potential dangers associated with Antibiotics agents are coming to be increasingly well-known however, many individuals remain confused or confused about the best time and when to remedies

Antibiotics agents. Resistance to antimicrobials is created by time and over using Antibiotics which increases the variety of microorganisms immune to medication.

Each of us is made up of trillions of tiny microscopic organisms. Some of which are helpful and essential to our health and health, while others cause harm when left uncontrolled. Every time you use Antibiotics that end up killing "great," delicate microorganisms inside your body, which have a an important task of reducing and adjusting harmful microorganisms. When taking anti-microbial drugs the immune microorganisms and germs can be left to grow and multiply faster, with no proximity to the amazing microscopic organisms you expect to combat them.

Anti-toxin resistance occurs when microbes undergo a change in an aspect that makes them immune to medications prescribed by professionals or synthetic chemicals, as well as other antibacterial experts. This poses a serious risk due to the fact that these drugs are intended to cure or stop illnesses, but they are ultimately useless and ineffective.

What is the best way for microscopic organisms to overcome Antibiotics and eventually become "immune"? There are a few ways in which this happens in which microscopic organisms build their capacity to kill the Antibiotics and others siphon Antibiotics from the body swiftly because of they tend to make them more powerful to do so, while others shift their target area to another location in the body.

Microorganisms that used to be susceptible to an anti-toxin could transform and change DNA and hereditary materials to create their own defenses. If a small number of microscopic creatures are immune to it, they would eventually be able to grow and replace all microorganisms killed off. These methods permit harmful microscopic organisms the ability in their reproduction and cause harm.

A judicious use of Antibiotics can help limit the spreading of resistance. Although antibiotics are needed every now and then to treat bacterial infections and certain dangerous maladies but they're not the most effective alternative, or the best treatment option for issues like viral infections that are common as well as the typical cold sore throat, the most common seasonal influenza. There are common steps that you can make to fight the influenza or cold, and solutions for sore throats that provide rapid relief, in addition to many other methods for treating sore throats and aches without Antibiotics.

In the present, a lot of useless Antibiotics agents are recommended each year to treat these kinds of ailments, even though they're not absolutely needed.

Perils of Antibiotic Resistance

Patients suffering from contaminations caused by tranquilizing immune microbes are generally at a greater risk of having more devastating clinical outcomes and possibly death. Patients with these conditions naturally spend more insurance benefits than those afflicted by similar microorganisms not immune from Antibiotics agents.

A gradual rise in protection against HIV medications was identified. From then on the further increases for protection by first-line treatments have been accounted for, which could mean using more expensive and extraordinary treatments earlier instead of later.

The moment is when we are seeing evidence of anti-microbial resistance in the almost endless and unaffected diseases there are. 2013 saw approximately 480,000 cases of multidrug-immune tuberculosis identified and confirmed in over 100 countries. This type of tuberculosis needs treatments that are more prolonged and more dangerous than active TB. Medical infection in the clinic are caused by highly immune microbes, for instance methicillin-immune staphylococcus aureus (MRSA).

All over the world there is protection against intestinal disease, HIV, increasingly Natural bacteria such as gonorrhea, respiratory tract infections and pneumonia, circulatory system illnesses and many more are recognized. Additionally, the spread or increase of Antibiotics resistant across the globe from region to region could impede significant progress in the control of many kinds of diseases.

The dangers of overusing Antibiotics agents do not end there. The main reason for using anti-microbials all the time is:

Connected to Higher Increase for Heart Disease

Here's a revealing statistic the use of Erythromycin was found to be a typical anti-microbial. It increases the risk of falling into the water from the heart up to 250 per cent!

This is associated with a higher Cancer Risk

Although Antibiotics agents themselves haven't identified as causing cancer in humans However, research has revealed an association between increased antimicrobial usage and a higher possibility, specifically bosom malignancy. It has been found that women who use Antibiotics agents more frequently - anywhere from just one to many times over the span of 17 years, appear to have a greater risk of malignant growth in the bosom. Researchers believe this is due to the effects of Antibiotics agents on the capacity of resistance as well as aggravation as well as digestion of estrogen as well as phytochemicals.

Makes a Higher Likelihood for Digestive Problems

"Great microscopic organisms" called probiotics are an enormous and important part of your digestive and immune related systems. They track the proximity of microscopic microorganisms that are harmful and aid in processing your food properly, taking supplements, and provide information to your brain in relation to your appetite, mental state and so on.

When you're deficient in microorganisms, due to taking Antibiotics which work to reduce the number of microorganisms in your digestive tract, you're unable to take in the nutrients you consume as well, and you're likely that you will experience signs such as the appearance of obstruction, swelling, or sensitivities and that's not even the beginning of the problem. There's a chance that you're more susceptible to nutritional deficiencies since you're unable to take in phytonutrients, nutrients and minerals , too.

Expands Risk for Allergies

Some studies currently indicate that the use of Antibiotics for children can increase the risk of hypersensitivities, asthma and dermatitis. Children are typically afflicted with colds, ear infections, sinus, and respiratory diseases. They receive immediately Antibiotics drugs to reduce the signs however, this can have negative effects.

A report that was recently that was published in Journal of Allergy and Clinical Immunology discovered it was the case that when Antibiotics were prescribed during the first year of a child's existence it was associated with an increased chance of developing the skin inflammatory condition and asthma. It was reported that 90% of respiratory infections are caused by viruses however, more than of 40 percent of anti-microbial treatments that are developed each year are approved for these contaminants, despite reality that Antibiotics do not have any effect on illnesses.

Young children also have an increased risk of developing food sensitivities, digestive issues and stomach-related problems especially in the event they do not eat supplements in their diet and aren't fed breastmilk. Studies have shown that many sensitive reactions that aren't favorable are caused by an unnatural level of intestinal vegetation, and the resulting poisonous quality that results due to poor absorption and poor eating habits.

The immune system is influenced by the mucous layer of the stomach's covering, and young people are prone to developing something called "gut as well as brain-science disorders" (GAPS). Although this could be a possibility for grown-ups too young people must an authentic GAPS diet, eat less carbohydrates and stay away from harmful substances or Antibiotics significantly more than adults, as their immune systems as well as their focal sensory systems are just developing.

Builds Cost of Health Care and Jeopardizes Current Treatments

Antibacterial resistance increases the cost of social insurance as it allows medical experts to employ increasingly complicated long-distance and non-immune treatments to combat illnesses which would in some way or in some way, be difficult to fight. When bacteria are ineffective against first-line medicines, more costly treatments have to be used for a longer period of duration.

This usually means a broader range of time in emergency clinics, increased medical services prices and a weight of money put on families, governments and social order. However, we are also placed at risk because antimicrobial defenses of various types (which is protection against microorganisms, but also different kinds of medications, too) can lead to counteraction and treatment of a range of Natural illnesses - such as the medical procedure, transfusions organ transplants, chemotherapy for malignancy and that's just the beginning of the iceberg more risky.

Forestalling Antibiotic Resistance

The introduction of Antibiotics within our system of care in the past 70 years was one of the most notable and life-saving developments to take place it is evident the problem is that in the present Antibiotics drugs are generally misused. While they've assisted many people over the years and are crucial treatment for certain bacterial infections such as pneumonia, and even real injuries, they're not ideal in treating viral infections hacks, or for preventing the flu or cold that is natural.

The most important thing is that every time you've taken Antibiotics previously you've killed off the horrible microscopic organisms that are causing your illness and yet, you've killed the good microbes, too. In order to naturally boost your gut, where the majority of the microorganisms are and help you support your immune system There are a few steps you can take.

Possibly Use Antibiotics When Necessary

If you're suffering from a debilitating condition and are visiting your primary doctor, discuss various treatments options and ask if the use of an antimicrobial is necessary. There could be other methods that are just as effective as anti-microbials, so don't think you'll require one or rely on your medical provider to suggest.

* Avoid taking Antibiotics to treat asthma-related side effects, regular hypersensitivity consequences, or viral diseases such as a stomach infection, or influenza. Use antibiotics only when absolutely necessary and only to eliminate all bacterial infections under control to avoid the obstructing of antimicrobials.

Don't share antimicrobials, and don't keep Antibiotics to take in the near time after you've been completely exhausted. Always dispose of any medications that remain after the treatment has been completed.

* Follow Antibiotics bearings in solution with care Don't miss doses and be serious about dosages or stop before completing the entire cycle.

Practice Good Hygiene to Prevent Spreading Germs

The most basic way to prevent bacteria and microorganisms that cause illnesses or contamination is to have the perfect family unit or workplace. It is important washing your hands thoroughly and take care to clean your kitchen and bathroom surfaces thoroughly, and refrain from going to work once you've cleaned up.

Use the usual antibacterial agents at home, such as essential oils, to keep bacteria and microbes without the use of chemicals or drugs that are synthetic. Anti-toxin oils that are commonly used can be included in essential oils, such as oregano as well as lemon oil and helichrysum essential oil. A large portion of these oils can also be used as alternatives for hypersensitivity that is characteristic. aid.

Making use of Natural methods is a safe bet in light of the fact that a link between synthetic antibacterial concoctions for business employed in household or household cleaning products and bacterial resistance has been observed in a few studies.

Increment Immunity Naturally Using Your Diet

Although it might appear as if it's difficult at first, or even completely getting rid of the majority of the starches, grains and sugars from your diet will help to replenish your gut and recharges your the defense-minded microorganisms. Even whole grains, are loaded with antinutrients and proteins like phytateand gluten, and lectin which are difficult to digest.

This is the reason for intestinal irritation and if you've had Antibiotics drugs a few times in your lifetime it is impossible to make it worse within the microbiome of your gut. Consuming a large amount of sugar within any form including grains or large amounts of starchescan help to control harmful microorganisms and allows the growth of more with no issue. Since these foods are separated into simple sugars within the stomach microorganisms are able to use them as fuel, which can overburden your immune system and renders you vulnerable to bacterial illnesses and infections.

Try growing grain breads or sandwich alternatives instead of the usual grains. Also, you can begin to use regular sugars rather than sugar.

Take Probiotics and Eat Probiotic-Rich Foods

Probiotics have been studied for their various medical benefits One of their main functions is to reduce the number of immune microorganisms and unimmune ones within the gut and increasing the number of good microorganisms. Their role in preventing the development of drug-induced diseases is currently being researched but it is now accepted that probiotics help improve gut health and immunity in individuals.

Probiotics refer to the "neighborly" bacteria that live in our stomachs and intestines that aid in the separation of our food items and in taking immune-boosting supplements to nourish our brain and organs. In reality the microscopic organisms (or those that are also types of yeasts and moulds) constitute an impressive 70-85% in our immunity system!

This is the reason why a better gut health condition is linked to fewer illnesses, including seasonal flu, asthma head colds, as well as UTIs.

Consume a high-quality probiotic supplement on a regular basis, particularly in the event that you've taken Antibiotics agents. It is also possible to consume rich in probiotics time to keep your intestinal verdure in check. To naturally restore the probiotics that reside in your digestive tract, I recommend that you consume a small portion of these probiotic foods frequently including Apple juice vinegar, processed dairy products (amasai, yogurt made from goat milk, kefir as well as refined yogurt that is made with cow's milk that is crude) and matured vegetables (sauerkraut as well as kimchi and kvass) as well as probiotic drinks (fermented tea, herbals from the territory and coconut Kefir).

Fortunately, these nutritious foods are becoming more accessible at the supermarket, even as details of the many benefits of probiotics in ensuring gut health get attention in the current media.

Devour "Earth's Antibiotics"

It is good news for us that there are many natural ingredients that could help reduce harmful microorganisms that are present in our bodies, lessen irritation and increase the proximity of defense microorganisms. Alongside eating probiotic-rich food Additionally, make it the effort to get enough gut-building, hypersensitivity-fighting food items that are "prebiotics." This includes items like asparagus, onions and a sluggish chicory root basic Jerusalem artichokes and the dandelion-colored greens. In addition, you should try to flush out commonly used antibacterial food items:

Chapter 11: The Immune System

Human immune systems is made up of two main components - the ambiguous immune system as well as the flexible (directed/explicit) resistance system. The two parts that comprise the immune system operate in tandem to shield the body from attacking and non-immune living forms like microorganisms, parasites, growths and diseases.

The First Line of Defense in the Anti-Disease System

The most important part of an individual's vulnerability (first layer of protection) is composed of two segments which are the mucous film and the skin (physical boundaries). If the outer skin hindrance is weakened then another layer of protection will be activated in the same manner. The most significant reason for the activation of the optional protection mechanism is irritation that is defined as a reduced redness, and it can grow wherever the life forms are present. It is also differentiated by a rise in the internal temperature (fever) and the proximity of discharges around the affected zone, and possibly the proximity of white plates within the pee.

A higher internal temperature (fever) is among the methods by which the body is able to maintain it's homeostasis (balance) with the intention that all synthesized responses within the body take place in a state of optimal efficiency, which is crucial to achieving an extreme level of health and wellness. A raised internal temperature can be a guide for destroying isolated living things.

Portions of the Primary Defense System

The diverse components of the fundamental security system comprise the:

Phagocytes are neutrophils and macrophages. Their main function is generally ingest and, in doing this, crush harmful pathogens. The process in which the phagocytes rise from the circulatory system and enters tissues to consume the attacking organisms is known as the process of phagocytosis. It is accomplished by the phagocyte recognizing the unimmune living form, taking it over and, as a result, eating the unimmune life form. Some microorganisms obscure their identities and cause confusion for phagocytes. However, the immune system can overcome this by blocking pathogens using Opsonins. These are proteins that supplement the immune system and are then able to provide "handles" for cells to bind to attacking pathogens, and by doing so, destroy them. In the event that certain pathogens are immune to these antibodies, the immune system at this point reacts by giving additional support - aid T cells release synthetic compounds that stimulate macrophages who then release additional harmful chemicals that can be deadly to the pathogens. Neutrophils can also penetrate the invading life-form's membrane by using defensins. Once the phagocytes are unable to ingest the invading organisms, they release toxic weapons to extracellular fluid, which is then used to pulverize these pathogens. Neutrophils destroy themselves while they are eliminating pathogens, but macrophages are able to continue pulverizing unwanted substances.

Common Killer Cells are found in the circulatory system , and in they are found in the lymphatic system. These cells are able to lyse, and thus destroy disease cells as well as infection-contaminated body cells prior to when the immune system turns on. They're part of a group of cells known as massive lymphocytes that are granular. They are capable of destroying a variety of distant immune cells and other life forms. They are ambiguous in what they're concentration on. Executioner cells that are characteristically able to kill harmful cells by entering them, and then triggering a specific cell passing (otherwise known as the process of apoptosis). They also emit chemical compounds that are solid and can accelerate the body's response to provocation.

Aggravation is part of the vital immune system. It's triggered by external trauma to body tissues, or as a result of severe heat (bringing about the consumption of) and substances that cause irritation to the skin, or from infections, parasites and microorganisms. The fiery reaction has several effects including the counteraction of the spreading of disease, the removal of dead cells as well as annihilated pathogens, and a heightened awareness for the immunity system, and creation of repair of cells and tissue. It begins with a substance alert. Synthetic compounds are released into the extracellular liquid they are released from injured or targeted cells. They can also be stimulated by the emergence of certain proteins in blood (histamine reaction). Macrophage cells (and various other tissues) possess unique capabilities for location that are in a position to trigger your immune system. The second effect of aggravation is the enlargement of the veins surrounding the area of the infection, which allows more bloodstreams into the region that accelerates fast healing. The tissues surrounding the veins are also becoming more permeable, in light of the transfer of immune system cells in a much faster manner towards the body part affected by the. Exudate results result of the increased development of blood cells and cells in the zone affected which results in a decrease in expansion. The liquid may press against nerve endings, which causes the pain reaction. Phagocyte assembly occurs due to the aggravation of the animal, and they are wiped out.

The Secondary Response System

The adaptive (or Secondary) Part of an individual's invulnerability the body's immune response, which can be acquired throughout the lifetime of exposure to various life forms that attack. The multi-faceted resistance system activates following the rapid response of the crucial immune system and is more than the basic defense against infection. The theory behind vaccination is that it's triggered through the inherent exposure of an infected or dead pathogen and the resultant effect on the body's immune response, is that it produces antigens that are specific to the pathogen. can be found within the resistant system.

The immune system's auxiliary and versatile is focused on the resistance to various creatures and their enactment causes the body respond to and destroy specific pathogens it is modified to fight. It prevents the spread of infection by similar living organisms. The secondary immune system has been activated without the person remaining alert. They could experience mild disturbances for a few hours or less this is due to the alternative immune system that kills an apparent pathogen.

Vaccination programs are essential in helping to prevent the spread of a variety of illnesses because they provide a targeted an all-encompassing response to counteract the effects of some harmful diseases. If the immune system is modified to a certain degree, it can destroy any pathogens it was recently exposed to. This immunity auxiliary focusing on susceptibility is able to put aside some effort to develop, which is why vaccine programs are extremely effective to prevent infections.

Immune System Stimulants

Many are in search of immune system stimulants or an immune-boosting system. It is why we offer the following information and helpful tips and strategies to help people protect themselves from the effects of colds, infections and bacterial infections. This article will focus on an overview of the importance of botanicals, herbs and other plant substances that could be considered to be an immune system stimulant that is commonplace but this is not in any in any way, form or manner an exhaustive overview. Researchers, specialists and scientists are always looking for new information and identifying new immune system stimulants that can be used to combat disease.

A complete immune system must begin with excellent wellbeing capabilities. When we were children we were instructed that we wash our hands after eating, but perhaps not before touching our faces. No matter what is your immune system stimulant it is likely to contract a bug or infection on the off chance you do not wash your hands prior to when you get in contact with your mouth, face eyes or nose.

The next significant step in the strengthening of your immune system is proper nutrition. A nutritional C supplement, which is the most natural stimulants for your immune system does not provide enough. If you're not getting enough calcium, or possibly magnesium, in that case the cells in your body are likely to not be able to absorb the nutritional element C. If the situation is that you consume an iron booster, however it isn't one that is a vitamin C supplement then the cells in your body are likely to be unable to store the iron. Minerals and nutrients work together. As part of the immune system, a complete multi-nutrient is more beneficial than a single nutrient boost by itself. Each day, multi-nutrients also ensure that you are receiving enough nutrients. We do not usually consume the right foods in the right proportions every day. Multi-nutrients protect against inadequate food intake and common resistance system stimulant.

You must get enough rest to allow the systems of your body to function effectively. The next thing to consider to strengthen your immune system is getting a sufficient evening's sleep. The research has confirmed that our mothers knew: the majority of people require at least 6-8 hours of rest every night for optimal well-being. Anything that could hinder an uninterrupted night of sleep with a predetermined schedule need to be treated prior to other immune system stimulants are able to function in a way that is appropriate.

As of now, we have a great health propensity as well as a daily multi-nutrient that provides an underlying restorative strengthening system. There are two things that must be avoided in order to benefit from this immune-system stimulant as well as a complete resistance fortifying system; smoking and stress. Although pressures that are transient, like such as taking part in sports or managing a sudden risk, releases synthetic compounds into the body. They provide a brief boost to the immune system Numerous studies have proven that constant pressure, which comes due to high weight work, a discordant relationship, or a variety of other factors that affect immune system response, can be a deterrent. If you're unable to alleviate the endless anxiety in your life, you'll have a requirements for an innate immune system stimulants that are resistant like plants and herbs are more important. If you smoke, C's nutrient is taken away from your body. It is inevitable that you will cause upper respiratory infections. The immune system of your body is enmeshed trying to counter the negative effects of smoking cigarettes and so efforts to build an immune system that is resistant will probably not work.

Everyone can benefit from resistance stimulants to the system, but people who work or live in an emergency hospital or nursing facility, people who interact with patients generally, have children at school, students in understudies and even those who eat out as frequently as they can are exposed to various distinct diseases and are in greater chance of developing illnesses. Stimulant to the immune system as well as the whole immune system are crucial for people with these particular conditions.

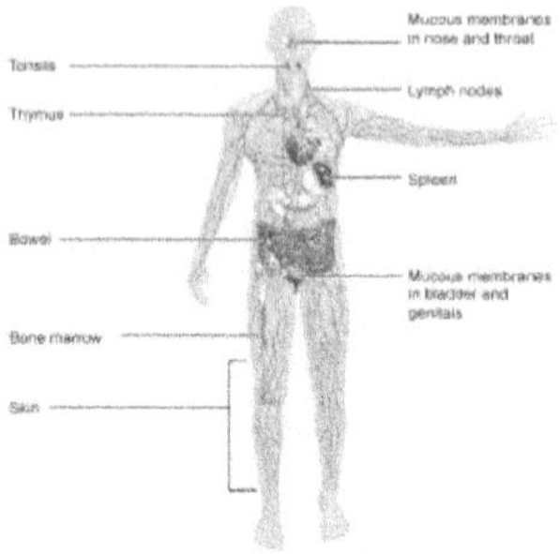

Resistant system stimulant with Beta Glucans, found in the cell dividers of oatmeal, grain, yeast and consumable mushrooms, as well as other plants, are the subject of a variety of scientific and clinical studies. One study showed that people who took these stimulants to the immune system had an increased number of T-cells that were assistants through the circulatory system. Aide T-cells are a specific type of white platelets that detect diseases and other things that aren't a good fit within the body. They tell the executioner T-cells how to eliminate the things. Beta-glucan supplements can be an important component of a complete resistance strengthening system.

An immune system stimulant like this herbal Andrographis Paniculata or AP for short could also be an important component in strengthening the immune system. AP has a history that is filled with the use of traditional Chinese treatment for the treatment of cold, contamination or fever as well as aggravation. Researchers studying herbs used in conventional medicine have shown that AP may be beneficial in the treatment of influenza, through reducing recovery time and the risk of causing discomfort. Although some herbs used as an immune system stimulant could be fatal when used over a longer period of time, AP has been appeared in animal studies to have a low or none of the toxic qualities.

Components of the Immune System

The immune system is comprised of a variety of parts that work to defend the body against intruders. The most important components that make up the immune system are the bone marrow as well as the thymus. The bone marrow plays a crucial role for the immune system as all of the platelets of the body (counting B and T lymphocytes) begin in the bone marrow. B lymphocytes are kept in the bone marrow and grow and grow, while T lymphocytes migrate to the Thymus.

The thymus is a bilobed organ that is located over the heart and behind the sternum and in between the lung tissue. The thymus only moves through pubescence. At the point of pubescence, it slowly shrinks, and is replaced by connective tissue and fat. Thymus is responsible to deliver the hormone thymosin that aids in the development and development of the T cells. In the thymus T cells grow, acquire specific antigen receptors, and then separate into helper T cells and T cells that can be cytotoxic. Different proteins are communicated to the T cell's surface. Thymus cells will have produced every T cell that meets an individual requirement by pubescence.

When the T and B lymphocytes are formed in the bone marrow and thymus after which they, at that stage, migrate to lymph hubs and spleen , where they remain until the immune system has been activated. Lymph hubs are located throughout the body. The spleen can be found within the left upper region of the midriff. It is located behind the stomach and below the stomach. The main function for the spleen the ability to channel blood. Red platelets that are solid and sluggishly move through the spleen. However the fact that damaged red platelets are sifted by macrophages (huge white platelets have experience in soaking in and taking care of cell flotsam, jetsam, pathogens and various non-essential substances found in the body) inside the spleen. The spleen serves with capacity for white platelets and platelets. The spleen assists the immune system by separating microorganisms which can cause disease.

In addition to the lymph hubs and spleen, mucosal associated lymphoid tissue (MALTs) and the gut-related lymphoid tissue (GALTs) perform a major role within the system of immunity regardless of their being thought to be the most important component that is part of the lymphatic system. MALTs are lymphoid tissues that are found throughout the body that have mucosa such as eyelids, digestive organs the skin, nose, and mouth. They are home to macrophages and lymphocytes that guard against pathogens attempting to enter the body. GALTs are lymphoid tissue found in the submucosa and mucosa of the digestive tract, tonsils, nutritional supplements and patches of Peyer's in the small digestive tract.

Immune Cells

Numerous cells collaborate in a significant way as part in the naturally (vague) and flexible (explicit) immunity system. Check out the section "Natural as opposed to Versatile Immune Reaction" for more information on an immune response that is natural and adaptable. Immune cells are again referred to as white platelets, or leukocytes.

Granulocytes are a type of leukocyte which has cells with granules containing chemical substances. Neutrophils and basophils as well as the eosinophils are a few types of the granulocytes. Neutrophils are thought of as experts to help the immune system that is inborn. The macrophages and the neutrophils circulate in the blood and reside within tissues, looking for problems. Both cells can "eat" microscopic organisms and converse with other immune cells in the event that there is a problem.

Cells belonging to the multi-faceted resilient system (likewise known as immune cells) have an immune function through an increase. Natural executioner lymphocytes and B lymphocytes are examples effector cells. In the case of T lymphocytes destroy pathogens the cell-intervened response. They release antibodies that aid in the development of an immune response. The effector cells are involved in the destruction and destruction of cancerous growth.

Non-effector cells are antigen-introducing cell (APCs such as dendritic cells as well as administrative T cells. myeloid-determined macrophages that are related to tumors, as well as silencer cells. Non-effector cells aren't able to be the sole cause of tumor-related passing. Non-effector cells hinder the immune activities of effector cells. In malignancy, these cells allow tumors to grow.

The reason for immune system weakness

Most of the time the immune system defends the body from infection. Yet, a handful of individuals have a weak resistance system, which could cause them to be more susceptible to illnesses.

White platelets, antibodies and other segments, like lymph hubs and organs are the components of the immune system of the body. Many scatters can weaken the immune system and lead the person to be immune compromised. The condition, known as immunodeficiency, is a range of mild to severe is present at birth or occur due to natural factors which are:

* HIV

* some malignancies of particular types

* malnutrition

* Hepatitis C virus

* some medications for clinical use

Every now and then the issue of immunodeficiency can become mellow to the extent that a person may not be aware of it for a significant amount of time. At other times the situation becomes more severe and causes an individual to be exposed to infections for a long time.

Take look at the consequences of a weak immune system. Then, suggest some steps that people could take to boost the chances of remaining strong.

A weak immune system

The primary consequence of a weak immune system is that it is more susceptible to illness.

Someone with a weak resilient system is likely to suffer from more infections every often than other people, and the symptoms could become more severe or difficult to manage.

The people who suffer from this condition could develop a disease which a person who has a stronger immune system wouldn't get.

The most common infections that people who have a weak immune system typically face are:

* pneumonia

* Meningitis

*bronchitis

* Skin contaminations

These infections can recur an increased frequency.

Other indicators of a non-power resistive system could include the following features:

* autoimmune disarranges

• inflammation in the internal organs

* Blood clutters or anomalies For example, weakness

* digestive problems, such as lack of craving, loose bowels and stomach squeezes

* deferrals of growth and formative development in infants and children

People with a weak immune system could discover a way to increase their odds of being healthy and avoiding a distance from illnesses.

Good cleanliness

Perhaps the easiest way to help someone who has a weak resistance system to stay strong is to practice maintaining a clean and tidy environment that includes washing their hands frequently. It is suggested to wash your hands on the occasions that follow:

* prior to, during, and following making suppers and bites

* Before eating

* After cleaning nasal mucus, wheezing or hacking

* prior to and following treating a cut , or any other open wound on the skin

* following contact with someone who's sick

* after using or helping an infant use the bathroom

* after changing the diaper

* following contact with a creature or a waste product or food source

* After contacting trash

The practice of washing your hands regularly can reduce the severity of ailments. Hand washing can reduce the incidence of loose bowel syndromes by 58 percent among those with weak immune systems.

Hand washing with water and cleanser can aid in ensuring children are safe and minimize the number of people who die from pneumonia or diarrheal illnesses among children younger than five years old.

Stay away from people who are completely exhausted

Immune systems that are weak should avoid becoming too close to any person suffering from an illness or cold. Diseases, infections and other irresistible illnesses can be transmitted from person to an individual via close contact. They may also spread via the water beads one throws in the air whenever they wheeze or hack.

It's not easy to keep a distance from people with a medical condition. However, anyone who has a weak immune system must remain at a safe distance from any close contact like hugging or kissing an unwell person until the sickness has gone away. Also, they should refrain from serving food or drinks to the person.

Sterilize the family unit's objects

Germs that may cause illness can be found on certain surfaces of the home, such as doors, handles as well as remotes. A person can cut down on the amount of germs which reside in these areas by cleaning the area regularly.

The majority of specialists recommend that the majority of people are awake and up-to-date with their vaccinations.

However, they can cause someone with a weak or compromised immune system to delay or decline certain shots.

If the transient illness or medication is responsible for the weak immune system, one could be able to acquire the antibody after the condition is gone or after they've stopped the treatment.

Examples of antibodies that doctors may recommend deferring or keeping an appropriate distance from include:

* MMR antibody for measles, mumps and rubella

* live influenza antibody

* MMRV antibody, which is part of the MMR immunization with the varicella (chickenpox) immunization

* rabies immunization

However those with a weak immune system must ask an expert to determine if antibodies they are allowed to carry and follow the recommendations of the specialist. Immunizations are a way to prevent one from being truly sick.

Oversee the pressure

Stress can affect the immune system and leave a person immune to disease.

Certain research shows that a person who is under a lot of stress is likely to fall sick.

Patients with a weak immune system must be able to cope with pressure. Strategies that can reduce and manage pressure include:

* Yoga

* Meditation

* massages

* spending time looking for leisure activities

Rest enough

According to The National Sleep Foundation, lack of sleep also affects the body's immune system , as does stress. Lack of sleep can affect the normal creation of white platelets, which is an essential part of the body's immune system.

As per the CDC the CDC, adults should concentrate on at a minimum 7 hours of sleep each day. Newborn children and young ones require someplace between eight and 17 hours of sleep based on their age.

Get a revigorating and healthy eating routine

A healthy and well-balanced routine of eating can enhance the overall health of a person.

If you have a weak or immune system, experts generally suggest eating a diet high in organic and vegetable foods, which can provide lots of nutrients.

If the person is immune compromised like, for instance, because they're under malignant growth treatments A doctor might suggest the patient to discover a method to avoid foodborne illnesses.

They could be:

* Washing all the soil-borne products the soil prior to stripping them

* Avoiding meats cooked to the point of being uncooked as well as eggs, fish, and other meats.

* refrigerating nourishment quickly

* opting for sanitized juices, and dairy products over nonpasteurized products

Perform your exercise routine regularly

Exercise is a natural way to keep your body well-maintained. While it is also a great way to strengthen the body, it also helps the body release endorphins which decrease the feeling of anxiety. However those with weak immune systems should be aware not to push themselves too in a way that could degrade the immune system.

As a result, people with weak immune systems could want to stay away from exercise:

* when it is too strong a force

* every now and then

* to stretch out the time in which you can rest

Consider taking steps to improve your skills.

Certain minerals and nutrients affect your immune system. For instance, a person with a vitamin C deficiency may suffer from an insufficiency.

Minerals and nutrients that influence immunity include:

* vitamin A

* Vitamin D

* vitamin E

* iron

* Folic acid

* zinc

It is recommended to obtain the supplements through diet sources whenever feasible but should the test results show that enhancements could help in reducing susceptibility. an array of supplements, such as multivitamins, can be purchased in health shops or on the internet.

The resistance system is a complex arrangement of organs and platelets, and protects the body from harmful bacteria that could cause illness. In the event that one feels that they are frequently and again afflicted with infections and infections, they could have weak immune systems. A person with a weak immune system may be able to make small strides in their home to stay healthy and increase their immunity.

Chapter 12: Why Healing Naturally

People seek natural remedies also known as home remedies or common fixes, for their ailments due to the fact that the medicines are created using common fixings such as herbs, plants, soil, and fixings easily found in any house. Home remedies do not use brutal synthetic chemicals, are cost-effective and generally they don't cause any problems. The majority of people also like making an item that is useful to use rather than buying expensive prescription drugs which may cause dangerous symptoms.

From the beginning of history have relied on traditional cures prior to the advent of modern medication and synthetic drugs. Many common diseases are treated with remedies that have fixings in the kitchen of your home.

The research has revealed a huge variety of mending substances found in the foods we consume each day. The experts at driving schools discovered that the naturally present nutrients contain the healing power to treat the most basic ailments, without a chance of reactions, and without having to pay the enormous cost of prescription drugs. Home remedies work quickly and safely and are generally beneficial for people who utilize them.

To make your own home remedies at your own home, all you need is the knowledge of how to make use of the most effective remedies and someone who can show or explain to you the most effective method to implement the standard treatments. There are a variety of books written on the subject and many websites with noteworthy Natural remedies.

Herbs, flavors, and fresh food items can be extremely effective for treating a variety of conditions ranging from minor discomforts to illnesses. Costly Antibiotics are extensively used nowadays, and in all likelihood they can, for the major part, be cured by regular treatments. The Antibiotics are naturally effective because they kill the microscopic organisms. Unfortunately, they also kill beneficial or amicable greenery, causing the body to require more time to recover that would have been required in the event that the Antibiotics agents not been employed.

Natural remedies are usually effective to treat minor infections as well as enhancing the body's immune system for be more likely to fight of various ailments like male pattern hair loss, skin break out flaws, dandruff and breakouts. advanced healing and repair of the throbbing, pain, and wounds and toxins.

It is possible to use home remedies to make your own mouthwash. It is a great way to rinse your teeth to prevent gaps and natural gum sickness. You can create a homemade solution to fix stomach-related problems, such as the stoppage, the runs, as well as acid reflux. Use a homemade solution to an assuage technique and speed up recovery from this winter's cold virus. Make a unique wash that soothes or calms sore throats. It is possible to mix distinctive throat rinses which can be used for treatments for asthma.

Regular cures aren't only effective to treat ailments in the inside, but, they can also be used as a chemical for treating skin problems that appear outwardly such as wrinkles and skin inflammation. Use natural solutions to fade the appearance of ageing spots or describe your remedy to lessen stretch marks and varicose veins. As a regular splash can help in removing out dermatitis or eliminating microscopic organisms that have accumulated in slices and scratches to prevent contamination or recoup annoyances.

If you are looking for a specific solution to your specific problem You will discover that there are a variety of proven remedies at home to treat a variety of common ailments. You can look into diverse solutions that are specific to those that work best for your specific condition. There is no need to depend on medications that could harm your body and may cost you lots of money to treat each one of your illnesses with home remedies that utilize distinctive ingredients, flavors, and foods can be found in the kitchen counter that puts aside money and can benefit your body.

Advantages of natural antibiotics

No matter if you're healthy or simply want to be healthier Natural antibiotics can be used. If you consider water to be unreasonably simple to drink natural antibiotics can be an effective alternative. Be sure to drink at the minimum five cups a day to reap the many health benefits. There are many medical benefits of drinking natural antibiotics but here are the top seven reasons you should consume these:

To Lose Weight

In order to get fit, using herbal antibiotics is a common theme. The reason antibiotics are effective in weight loss is mainly because they improve the digestion of your body and consequently enhance the health of your heart, improve blood circulation and ultimately lower the cholesterol levels. In green antibiotics there is a substance that many refer to as cell-reinforced catechins. These research has shown that they aid in the consumption of fat.

Forestall Cancer

Did you know that Japanese people who consume antibiotics are less prone to malignant growth of the lung? Truthfully, natural antibiotics can help treat heart problems as well as strokes and prevent certain illnesses!

Fix Stomach Disorder

If you're suffering from stomach problems, you can have try drinking herbal antibiotics right after wrapping the meal. Natural antibiotics allow your stomach to digest the food efficiently by reducing the acidity.

Better Immune System

Natural antibiotics can strengthen your body as well as your immune system, ensuring to prevent the spread of the flu or any other lung disease. With more well-balanced cells in your body, you can recuperate and repair the hurt cells more quickly.

To Reduce Stress

If you feel that your life style and work is a bit gruelling So why not take a look at natural antibiotics? It's extremely unwinding and definitely effective in reducing the pressure.

Better Sleep at Night

Natural antibiotics can aid in promoting to sleep. If you're having trouble sleeping in the evening, take a the chance to drink some natural antibiotics 30 mins before you head to bed.

More beneficial than coffee

Herbal antibiotics are less caffeinated and are an excellent alternative to those who are healthy enough to be aware of the need to stop tooth decay. Did you know that antibiotics are mainly comprised of the same amount of fluoride as well as a couple of particular Antibiotics that help prevent gum diseases and the formation of plaque?

How do you treat infected areas naturally

When you regularly visit the emergency department and are examined for the signs of bacterial diseases and you realize it's a kind of contamination caused by microorganisms, which will result in negative consequences for you. In any event, it is evident that a significant portion of us aren't thinking clearly about this illness. What is a bacterial illness and the best way to deal with bacteria are among the most often asked questions that people often think of when they are confronted with the problem. In all likelihood there are numerous posts that provide information and clarification on the bacterial problem, but they could not include all important information.

The text will provide you with the most information that can be expected in terms of its definition, manifestations and signs as well as medicines and other. It's unfortunate in the event that you do not read the text because it's beneficial to you. This is the best time to take the chance to look over the bacterial infection.

All Facts About How to Treat Bacterial Infection Naturally

What Is Infection?

To fully understand the nature of bacterial infection and how to treat the bacterial diseases, it is important to understand the concept of microorganisms. Microorganisms are tiny, single-cell organisms that exist all over, regardless of the climate and the place. As you may have guessed microorganisms are visible all over the earth, in water, soil, and other areas. They also reside on and within many conveying areas including animals, plants as well as human bodies. In this way, they have specific effects on the conveyancing groups, actually. Despite the benefits that they bring such as the fact that they have vital functions for animals just like in nature microorganisms have been thought of as having a negative significance. The bacteria that cause the disease is a good example.

If you require a thorough understanding of the world from all the way from top to bottom, then you can click on and go through the specific research on microscopic organisms.

The majority of the term "bacterial infection" refers to the spread of destructive microorganisms that are found on or within your body. Food contamination, pneumonia as well as meningitis are just a number of illnesses caused by microorganisms. They are actually in three main shapes: pole-molded as well as helical and circular.

They're also divided in two types: gram-positive or negative. Gram-positive microscopic organisms possess cells with a thick divide, gram-negative organisms don't. The truth is, in the event you're assessed for the effects of a bacterial illness You may have come across various tests to examine the pattern of microbes. For instance, gram recoloring is a method of testing the efficacy of bacterial cultures using antibiotics is a possibility. This can help us decide the most effective treatment. It is generally recommended that we respond to the question of how to treat bacterial diseases.

The bacterial infection is an infectious disease, which means it could be transmitted from person to individuals through close contacts with the patients. Exposure to affected surfaces, the food items, water, just like wheezing or hacking are just a few examples. Furthermore, microscopic organisms may also cause a severe illness that can be treated quickly and continuously. The problem could last for a considerable time in all likelihood, for an actual existence, and an inactive illness that may not show any obvious symptoms or signs at first but can appear after a period of time. The symptoms of this current illness could vary from mild moderate, and even an extreme. In the most serious instances the condition can cause death for many people For instance, many people died because from bubonic plague. Black Death or bubonic plague.

Indications of Infection

In reality it's difficult to find the entire range of the signs and symptoms of bacterial illness. At this point, I could be able to provide you with the more Natural ones. The typical side symptoms of the bacterial illness include heaving, irritation squeezes, diarrhea, looseness of bowels as well as weakness, hacking and sniffling. Therefore should you suspect that you experience any of these side effects take into consideration how to deal with bacterial infection in the future, since you may begin to be suffering from the negative effects of it.

Particularly the case of bacterial contamination, it is separated in a variety of types of structures, which include microbes responsible for contamination of food and sexually transmitted diseases and many more.

Causing Food Poisoning

Here are some of the most common adverse effects that can be found in cases of bacterial illness found to be related to food contamination.

* Campylobacter jejune is a gastrointestinal illness which is often accompanied by a fever or other issues

* Escherichia coli (or E.coli for short) is a different type of diarrheal illness with side effects that include nausea, vomiting stomach spasms, vomiting, and nausea.

* Clostridium botulinum is thought to be potentially dangerous bacterium that produces neurotoxins that are ground-breaking.

* Salmonella is frequently accompanied by stomach spasms, fever and loose bowels.

* Listeria monocytogenes may cause an increase in fever, muscle throbs, and the looseness in the bowels. Particularly, elderly

people or pregnant women, as well as babies who have an immune system that is weak will likely experience negative effects of this condition.

* Last but not least the vibrio, which is a part of the runs. Sometimes the microbes that are present in an open wound may cause serious skin irritation, which could cause a significant problem when you do not receive the proper treatment at the right time.

Check out these Home Remedies for Food Poisoning and get Natural solutions to food poisoning.

Sexual Transmitted Diseases

This is an issue that is alarming that is why you are required to be aware of it.

* Chlamydia is a common problem in both individuals, and is caused through Chlamydia Trachomatis. This causes the possibility of irritation to the pelvis in the woman's uterus.

* Bacterial vaginosis is one among the transmitted sexual illnesses caused by microorganisms. It triggers an increase in pathogenic microorganisms within the vagina. It is believed to be linked with a variety of unhealthy health conditions as well as insufferable complications

* Gonorrhea result from Neisseria gonorrhoeae that can be found in two individuals.

* Syphilis is a different bacteria-related disease that affects both genders. The microorganisms Treponema pallidum is the primary cause of this condition. If it isn't treated properly this will result in an issue that is risky.

Other Bacterial Infection

* Otitis media refers to a disease that affects the ear's center that can result from an infection caused by a virus or bacteria and can be seen frequently in infants and infants.

* Urinary tract diseases are also a different kind of bacterial infection that is that affects kidneys, bladders and urethra.

The condition of the respiratory tract is caused by microorganisms, or infections. It includes sinusitis, bronchitis as well as sore throat.

Home Remedies on How To Treat Bacterial Infection

Although Antibiotics drugs are among the well-known treatment for bacterial infections however, there is a belief that they can trigger a variety of significant problems. In the end, we'll need to provide you with common methods of the best method to treat bacterial diseases.

Step-by-step instructions on how for treating Bacterial Infections Cranberry Juice

The consumption of Cranberry juice has been proven to be a powerful ingredient in the treatment of bacterial contamination and countermeasures, such as Escherichia Coli that affects the epithelium of the bladder. In particular, evidence indicates that this juice may be utilized to stop UTI in females but there isn't any evidence to support the claims of children.

If you think about it all things considered, cranberry juice is an excellent tip for the most effective way to fight bacterial naturally which is able to treat vaginal and urinary tract infections. The cranberry juice which isn't improved and can be used typically throughout the day to fight the harmful microorganisms that reside in our bodies. It is possible to use cranberry juice in a safe manner even for women who are pregnant to restore bacteria that have been contaminating. This is why it's prescribed to you in the event of possibility that you must discover how to treat bacterial infections with no antibiotics. As it is in the context of it being true that juice from cranberries is appropriate for kids however, its corrosiveness could make it less popular among the. The truth is the percentage of the juice that is intended to prevent UTI from children hasn't been determined at the moment. It's an unresolved problem.

Step by step directions to treat bacterial infections by using Tea Tree Oil

In January of 2006 an examination published via Clinical Microbiology Reviews, discharged the evidence of tea tree oils possessed an antibacterial effect. In reality, there are many studies which have proven the beneficial antibacterial properties of this common oil, regardless of the differentiators among their methods, the results are still extremely comparative and consistent. In spite of the fact this wonderful essential oil is renowned due to its antiviral as well as antibacterial capabilities and its antibacterial properties, it's extremely effective in fighting against a vast range of skin and vaginal illnesses caused by microorganisms.

The oil of tea tree, which can be applied to the skin safely or in your vaginal waterway and crushes the bacterial activities and, in all cases, is necessary to be weakened enough to ensure a secure distance from the dangers of consuming skin. Because this oil is extremely powerful and potent, it can be used for the purpose of reversing and preventing endless contamination. However, it doesn't cause any or symptom.

Aloe Vera for Bacterial Infection

Another option for the most effective way to treat bacterial infections is using Aloe Vera.

You are likely conscious, Aloe Vera is notable for its amazing effects on our hair, skin, and overall health. It also has a great track record in curing bacterial diseases and bacterial infections, which is not an amazing fact. In fact multiple studies have proven the properties that is present in Aloe Vera. For example The African Journal of Biotechnology distributed an examination that was conducted at an examination conducted by the University of Karachi in May 2020. According to this study, Aloe Vera was tried against both gram negative and gram positive skin infections that segregate. Furthermore, a favorable result was which showed that 95% of living things tested were gram positive and only 10% been gram-negative. The antibacterial properties were derived out of Aloe Vera extricate, as opposed in its leaves. Due to its beneficial properties for reducing and preventing bacteria, Aloe Vera is considered as the most effective method to treat bacterial diseases without Antibiotics. In addition, the remedy offers the ability to heal and restore, and it also assists you to lessen the impact of bacterial illness and reduce the risk of developing. Additionally, it is the case that it fights bacterial infections and inflammation, the gel of aloe can treat various ailments like inner disease, urinary tract , or vaginal illness. Aloe Vera must be considered as a viable solution on the most effective way to deal with bacterial infections when it is applied to the skin areas affected by it. Allow it to sit for a few minutes prior to washing off by using warm water. Another method you could try eating Aloe Vera juice that produces similar effects. In general, Aloe Vera does a great job of treating bacterial infections and, therefore, you should take into consideration using it if you experience issues like this.

There's a wide range of content on Aloe Vera along with its benefits to skin that you're attracted to You can look up "Aloe Vera For Wrinkles" or "Aloe Vera For Skin Whitening".

Garlic on how to Treat Bacterial Infection

You are able to put your trust in garlic because it's also a characteristic home remedy that has antibacterial properties. Garlic can be found in any kitchen, and is an most effective home remedy to treat many bacterial and contagious illnesses. The most effective and most effective method of treating bacteria is to eat 4 to 5 cloves of garlic each day. It is possible to chew and then swallow it. Another option is to take garlic in the form of cases. However this scenario, it is less persuasive than eating garlic on its own. If you aren't able to keep the freshly cut garlic cloves, then you could contemplate the causes of it however, we regardless, recommend consume it in a sloppy manner. Additionally, the tea of garlic is an alternative which is also regarded as the most natural remedy for most effective method to treat bacteria. Include one or two cloves of garlic in the boiling water and let it sit for a few minutes before tasting the tea. It's not that difficult to drink a glass of garlic tea, with the intention to put in some effort and time in it. Garlic tea can be an effective treatment.

Nectar - Effective Remedy For Bacterial Infection

You might have heard of the benefits of nectar in terms of health and magnificence , but perhaps you haven't thought of its antibacterial properties. The benefits of nectar that comes from nature differ with the aim to be discovered little by little. The truth is that nectar is an effective treatment for skin and respiratory diseases and cool affected regions all the while. Drinking nectar from nature along with a glass of warm water to ease and ease the sore, painful throat caused by a cut. In the event that there are open injuries cut, scratch or abrasions on your skin, the most effective technique to stop any dreadful microorganisms from gaining access to the cut is to apply nectar to the affected areas as the treatment.

Ginger

If you are required to look for diverse suggestions on the most efficient way to treat a bacterial infection You are not required to stay away from ginger. It is effective in treating respiratory and stomach issues. It cools your body and increase your blood flow. Therefore, ginger can help in reducing the amount of harmful microorganisms within your body. To ensure well-being of your respiratory system, it's recommended to drink ginger tea three or four times a day. You can also apply a gentle rub to your affected skin. In addition, by increasing blood flow, these lines , it will help by reducing the discomfort caused by the bacterial illness.

It's also apparent that ginger is among the top multi-utilitarian solutions for natural wellness conditions.

Lemon for Bacterial Infection

Lemon is a different home remedy which treats a myriad of infections caused by microorganisms especially respiratory diseases. Lemon helps in removing the bodily fluids that are accumulated within the respiratory tract. Additionally, drinking a lemon juice can also eliminate the microorganisms trapped within the mucous. So, lemon juice is essential on the list of suggestions for the most efficient treatment for bacterial infections.

Additionally, let us help you remember another important health benefit of lemons as well, which is the capacity to fight asthma and sensitivity due to the significant amount of vitamin C it has. If you're required to do further research then you can do so by following this link.

As you are probably aware the preparation of soft drinks is used for a variety of purposes, ranging from cooking to managing beauty and health. The step-by-step instructions for how to treat bacterial diseases by drinking a warming soft drink is one of the things we'd like to demonstrate in the following. Through an investigation on the antibacterial properties of sodium bicarbonate soft drinks was proven to have a remarkable antibacterial effect. Due to its capacity to regulate the PH parity of your body and skin making a home remedy for soft drinks can be used to treat a variety of ailments caused by microscopic organisms, such as for instance, respiratory infections and bacterial skin diseases, and intestinal tract diseases. In addition, if you mix one half teaspoon of prepared soft drinks into the form of a glass of water it could aid in treating stomach diseases and respiratory infections. Another way to use this staple of the kitchen on the most efficient way to treat bacterial diseases is to add the remedy to the tub of water that is tepid. The remedy can be used each day to flush and drenching professional.

Turmeric on How To Treat Bacterial Infection

Alongside ginger, turmeric can be also referred to as a reliable natural remedy for a variety of health issues. There are actually a lot of research studies that show the incredible effect of this element in terms of health and efficiency in general including the ability to fight against microorganisms' merits when considering.

Particularly, many people realize that turmeric is the most effective cure for tumors that can be dangerous. One possible explanation is that curcumin , a component of turmeric, is antibacterial, calm and cell-building properties. In addition, the use of the turmeric glue created by grinding turmeric, could be effective in treating skin infections caused by bacteria. It is recommended to apply the glue on the affected area in order to ease the effects. After several minutes then wash it off with warm water.

Apple Cider Vinegar

This is a major misunderstanding in the event that we fail to consider the important task of apple cider vinegar as the most effective way to treat bacterial infections without antibiotics. In reality vinegar generally and apple juice vinegar specifically has antibacterial and hostile to infection capability to fight the bacterial infection. A review published in a Med Gen Med article on May 30, 2006, revealed that using vinegar to combat diseases is crucial.

The most common ailments to treat through herbal

Homegrown is a great remedy for a variety of pain and help you to feel better.

Hypertension or High blood pressure

Hypertension, also known as hypertension, is the unspoken anti-ageing foe. It kills you with your essential supply of vitality, and is now moving towards death and complete destruction. The intricate nature of life forces the level of adrenalin in the blood to rise , which triggers the expansion in the rate of pulse. This is a kind of infection that can be an explanation for illness and as a result, without the prescribed medication of your doctor you could, in reality begin with your own home remedies for hypertension. This is certainly effective, causing you to feel relaxed and comfortable.

Amla also known as the alternative name is Indian Gooseberry is among the most effective home remedies to treat hypertension. Normally, if you could consume a spoon of juice from amla mixed together with nectar, it will that it will be a great way to monitor the degree of BP. It is also possible to try cayenne pepper to achieve this. You must drink warm water and one teaspoon of cayenne pepper. Drink this solution and you will feel much better. If your circulation strain is rising up, try having the 100g of lemon dissolved in with water . You should drink this as if you were clocking in an immediate relief from the weakness.

A mixture of garlic and tar could be considered as one of the most remarkable natural remedies to hypertension. Furthermore in the event you develop the habit of eating papayas on a an empty stomach, you could have the option to ease yourself out of this unusual situation. It is possible to make the cinnamon seeds, sugar, and Fennel seeds, and then crush them to store in a holder that is empty. Mix the mixture of one teaspoon into an ice-cold glass of water and drink it. Continue this process for a couple of days. Then you can check your results to observe the adjustments on the BP level.

A blend of onion juice and nectar is also effective to reduce the degree of hypertension. If you are able to take 2 tablespoons from this mixture normal, you could in actuality, return to your normal routine with vitality and fun. Garlic is regarded as one of the most effective remedies for hypertension that is available at home. You can use this common component to address issues like the solidification of blood vessels, high blood cholesterol and thrombosis. It is also possible to have watermelon as a form of treatment for hypertension.

Each day and night, you can take pleasure in what is known as fenugreek seeds. Take the seeds for about 10 days with water and notice how it performs in making you feel more relaxed and confident. Apart from drinking and eating and using a few natural remedies for hypertension, you should adhere to certain guidelines to stay healthy and healthy. In every instance, better to walk in shoes on the green grass. In any case, do this for between 15 and 20 minutes each day, and observe the results it brings. Your health is an asset all the time Therefore, you must to take every step to ensure it is protected and ensure its health.

Tonsillitis

Depends on the severity of the situation of tonsil stones Based on the severity of the stones, there are distinct remedies that may be attempted.

Certain of them can be treated at home, while other require a visit to a doctor's office. Fortunately, tonsil stones can be treated. an issue that responds to various medications within short time.

The main goal of the vast majority of methods of treatment is to flush out the stones, so that the body's natural processes would then be able to absorb and effectively eliminate the tonsil stones, without causing any harm to the tonsils in the proper way. In all instances the case of a medical emergency it could be necessary to use a device to remove the tonsil stones and the body out and out.

For home remedies to treat tonsil stones, watering your area is the most common method. This may include the use of mouthwashes, or even water that has been treated using salt.

The water system could involve the delivery of the liquid both through the mouth as well as through the nasal passages. This method is believed to successfully sandwich in the tainted area and then attack tonsil stones with two distinct angles. There are various flooding devices which can aid in this technique.

Another method of home treatment is to increase the amount of liquid. However, instead from the water system patients will use the motion of swishing to remove the stones, allowing them to pass across the entire system. In the meantime mouthwash or saltwater may be used for the rinse.

There are a few home-grown methods which incorporate garlic and other fixings, for instance. mixtures of herbs into an energizing combination that will help in removing the stones and begin healing the tonsils that have been contaminated too.

Toothache

Do you really believe that you're always suffering from that toothache? Do you not want to miss the chance of visiting the dentist? Have you tried a shot at the chance to end that horrible agony? Imagine a scenario where I would inform you that there was a simple solution to your problems. These strategies don't work on their own but they also work fast to help you return to your normal life that you lived.

People, in general do not have a chance to stopping toothache pain because they have no notion of the primary cause of the pain. The majority of toothaches are caused through irritation and disturbance of the central zone of the tooth, but it's not the primary reason. Toothaches can result from many angles, including cavities, food particles stuck in teeth, as well as physical damage due to a mistake. But, not every expectation is gone. There are methods available that have assisted other people and can also help you, without paying attention to the motive.

Here's a sample of the traditional techniques you should try first prior to attempting other methods. Cleanse your mouth using a little water to eliminate and excess nutrition that could be contributing to pain. Additionally, be sure to floss regularly (however be cautious because the area can be damaged). The elimination of anything that can cause discomfort is the first stage in stopping the toothache. After that, mix your mouth with saltwater (1 teaspoon per cup of water) and then murmur it in your mouth on a regular basis every two weeks.

If your toothache doesn't go away in the present try this simple and easy treatment. This method involves the use of clove oil.

Clove oil isn't expensive and difficult to obtain and can be used in conjunction with a discomfort prescription. Use clove oil and then plunge it into an q-tip. The area of the body that is hurt by using this q-tip. You should feel relief. It is also possible to apply clove oil using an unbleached cotton ball and take a bite of it in the area of discomfort.

Gum disease

It's not a surprise that drained gums can be found in 3 of four adults over 40 years of age. A lot of people deal with their teeth by keeping their teeth clean all often they can neglect their gums. When this happens, their gums could be continuously heated, and if untreated, they can lead to an extreme case of gum disease.

Gum disease can have conceivably real effects, which include the loss of teeth. However, before that happens, those with a swollen gum will typically experience gums that dripping when they brush or eat. If someone finds their gums draining properly they must discover a solution to the problem. This can be done using the remedies at home.

The most important thing to do when they observe the gums of their mouth are dripping is to floss and brush their gums and teeth naturally. Flossing is especially important because of its ability to eliminates tiny particles of food which are trapped within the tooth's middle that cause inflammation and the development of tartar. By flossing at any frequency, twice each day, you'll eliminate of the growth that has formed around the gum line, and gradually repair gums that are draining.

If you notice that there is a painfully growing gums, making flossing and brushing difficult try a toothpaste that is distinctive by a homegrown arrangement to soothe the gums. For instance peppermint oil, and tea tree oil are highly beneficial. A mouthwash that is distinctive that is made from myrrh or sage will aid in fighting against microorganisms.

There are various kinds of gums-draining treatment available in the local supermarket or at home. One is to make use of heating pop. This will help ease the discomfort that causes the gums to dry out. Because the heating soft drink is a chemical base it can assist in neutralizing the impact of microbes responsible for the increase. Simply mix heating pop with water to create glue, and then apply it on the area that is being heated.

Ginger is a different kind of gum treatment that drains the gums. It doesn't require a dentist and can be prepared at the kitchen at home. Ginger is well-known as a recuperative agent and is mixed with salt to create glue which can be applied safely on the gumline. This method should be applied a few times a day to get the optimal results.

Rinsing is another method to treat dripping gums. For this, make use of warm water, and then add one teaspoon of salt to the glass. Rinse it a few times throughout the day with warm salt water especially in the beginning of the day, and then around the time of sunset. This will allow your whole mouth to become healthier and more effective. This technique is best done with an unsweetened glass of Cranberry juice.

In addition to the above kinds of gum disease treatment that drains, those who are suffering from the signs of gum disease could also discover that increasing their consumption of fresh natural foods including vegetables and fruits, as well as in general, nutrient-C aids in relieving gums that are draining. Vitamin C is a great way to get rid of all kinds of harmful substances like microorganisms and increase the flow of blood into the gums. Try your hand at eating. However, as a new , natural substance as might be expected, it will help to reduce the microscopic bacteria that reside in your mouth. It will also aid the healing process of your gum line.

Skin breakout

Home remedies for acne breakouts can be done easily at home. And you aren't required to fret about numerous visits to the dermatologist , or incur the huge cost of going to them. In addition, some of the treatments you receive when visiting the dermatologist may be challenging to. Natural remedies can be considered as easy treatments that can be consumed during a meal or by buying a topical cream which can be used every day for two hours. If you decide to use remedies that are made at home to help treat breakouts on the skin, be sure you do your research to find out exactly what the ingredients are likely affect your body, or interact to other medications you could be taking. These remedies are harmful for women that are expecting, suffer from diabetes, kidney issues, or and diabetes, therefore speaking to your physician is in all situation the best option. One thing to keep in mind when using an organic supplement is certain herbs perform well in other cases, but you don't see any improvement. It is important to find the right herbs that will work for you, and this will require a lot of effort and energy. Some of the herbs that people have observed to be effective include Milk Thistle, Red Clover, Licorice Root, and Echinacea.

Milk Thistle helps to protect and regenerate the liver. In the body, poisons which can drain your liver cause the formation of poisons that aren't made in the digestive organs but in your pores will be clogged, leading to skin breaking out.

Red Clover is a vegetable as well as soy is a source of phytoestrogens which are synthetic plant substances very similar to human estrogen. Red Clover has been utilized to treat certain ailments, for instance, bloodstream, diabetes menopausal, menopausal, elevated cholesterol osteoporosis and cancerous growth, and inflammation of the skin. Research suggests the fact that once estrogen levels rise your mental state alters, your hormones even out, and the production of oil slows down.

Licorice Root is mitigating. It helps to stop growing down, as well as treating the signs of bumps that are red and raised.

Echinacea has been used for treating influenza and colds due to its power to immunity. A healthy immune system allows you to fight off microorganisms as well as illnesses that cause your skin to breakout.

Skin inflammation

Eczematous disorders can be characterized by a broad range of signs. It is a sign of irritation that can be followed by the appearance of redness. The skin becomes flaky whenever there is a constant scratching because when dermatitis strikes the skin, it becomes dry. It also causes discomfort and irritation can develop and eventually develop. These symptoms can persist for a considerable period of time and can even last for days. Atopic dermatitis that is persistent can remain on the skin for an extended amount of time, sometimes for months, if not addressed. Treatment with elective medications using herbal remedies is a key element to healing. It is important to research ways to reduce inflammation of the skin using natural remedies!

Relieve dermatitis when the rashes appear, using the sandalwood glue and blend of camphor. To reduce the severity of irritation blueberry extricates are transformed to cream, and then shark ligament could be used. To clean the affected part with pine tar, you can use a cleanser. Nutrient E removes toxins from enhancements and will help to keep a safe distance from irritations and also reduce it.

To treat oral prescriptions, dietary supplements that are rich in tomato juice and zinc aid in boosting the immune system's capacity to combat allergens that are the reason of Allergic Contact Dermatitis. To combat two kinds of treatment, you could make a mixture of these plants to create an emulsion of spearmint leaves, dandelion leaves and very little drop of olive oil. It's a good moisturizer that helps in hydrating the skin. Use this instead of other products for restorative use available on the market to ward off free radicals utilized in the creation of these excellent products. Natural creams are able to repair the skin's outer layer.

If the skin appears flaky or layered or layered, it is essential to shed the layers and an abundance of nuts that absorb water could be a great cleansing scour. Cleansers for the body available have synthetic ingredients and when used in the process of shedding the affected part they may also trigger skin inflammation as they strip continuously the epidermis can affect the dermis. Following shedding, it's best to keep your skin hydrated and well-hydrated especially on the off possibility of living in a country that experiences difficult winters. The lotions and creams used in business contain fragrances that could harm your skin and cause more skin irritation. Virgin Coconut Oil can be employed as an alternative. It has lauric corrosion, which aids in rehabilitating.

Chapter 13: Boost Your Immune System With Herbal Medicine

Herbs that boost your immune system can help keep your immune system in good shape and well-balanced (balance is key) and can ward off the harmful pathogens that harm your health and simultaneously enhancing the more accommodating ones. There's a unique remedy or herb for every illness or problem we confront every day. It is our responsibility to discover the remedies that have been used successfully over a number of years, just like the present all-encompassing medicine provides us with these are just an answer to keep us healthy and healthy for our entire lives.

The Immune System Supplement boost your immune system, and aid in equalization. Regarding your overall health there is no higher concern than keeping the primary line of protection against infection (your body's immune system) functioning at a high level to protect your body from the ravages of infections, germs and bacterial toxins you interact with every single day. There are many amazing herbs to help maintain the balance of your immune system, just like foods that boost your immune system to help you stay healthy and positive as you journey through the complexities of life.

Chapter 14: Garlic - A Powerful Antibiotic

With the increasing number of reports on immune microorganisms with antimicrobial properties, it is the ideal opportunity to study the possibility of trying to repair the body naturally first. Although typical cures should not substitute for the guidance of an expert in the field however they may help to transform any potential infection into something that is more sensible when applied initially implemented.

The battle against stomach and sinus issues by taking oregano oil. Take oregano oil in your mouth it is formulated to deal with stomach related issues. This includes a variety of food borne illness, breathe in oil and gently exhale to lessen and possibly eliminate the effects of sinus diseases.

* Pour the oil into a mug made of earthenware or a tiny glass bowl. Then, heat using the microwave (or in a dish placed on an oven stove) until the oil has a good simmer.

* Sit on the bowl or mug and cover your head out with the towel. Keep towel open toward mug or bowl.

* Breathe deeply and inhale oil Close your eyes to avoid causing trouble.

Take a bite of the Natural cold as well as other common microbes, yeasts and parasites and infections by eating garlic. As a method of fighting MRSA The garlic plant is the most effective remedy for a deep-rooted many diseases.

Squash one smashed clove of garlic using the garlic press. Make sure you do this on the bowl or on a towel to extract any liquid.

* Cut the garlic into small pieces with a blade , and let it sit for to rest for 5 minutes prior to releasing.

Reduce the duration of the normal cold by taking Echinacea. The ongoing study has revealed that Echinacea users reduced the natural duration of their cold by 26%..

* Take three doses of Echinacea during the flu and cold season to reduce the chance of being sick and also to reduce the length.

* Drink tea with Echinacea on the off chance that you lean toward over-supplementation.

Protect yourself from MRSA or other skin infections by using turmeric. When you apply it to the contaminated cut or bubbles, turmeric can be thought of to work as an amazing antibacterial agent.

* Mix two pieces of turmeric and one of water that has been refined. Mix well until it forms a glue.

* Spread glue over the damaged area and let it dry.

Stop the spread of infections like strep and skin disorders by using nectar.

Simply apply the product to the affected skin and allow it to sit upon the surface.

Garlic is a profitable crop that you could cultivate in pots. In fields , you divide the plants by lines, one foot apart so that you can walk between them.

However in holders, you can simply walk through the outer edges of the plant, which means the cloves could have just four creeps on each pathway.

In the event that you try to purchase garlic, you'll be able to see the significance of cost. When you consider that each clove will produce somewhere between 10-15 cloves, it should be extremely useful from a purely a practical point of view for customers who want organic produce.

The most efficient method to grow garlic is to create it.

How do you create these? Put cloves in the ground across your garden and let them move as they please. This will aid in the growth of your various plants. To grow them into harvests, it is recommended to use raised beds. For instance the trash can could be a good raised bed in the event that you perforate the bottom and cut it down to about 9 inches tall. If you're cautious you can get 3 or 4 rings of each container, each 9 inches tall for the holding dividers that you will need for those raised beds.

Each ring can produce around 25 bulbs, and there could be many cloves within each bulb.

The rings should be filled with compost mixed in with a bit of dirt. It has to be diminished and abundant.

In a few years after that, you'll have your own collection. At first you can buy bulbs from a local producer or from members of a natural group can swap bulbs. Garlic bought from shops is naturally sprinkled with flowers to prevent the growth of these bulbs. In addition, purchase your supply locally. As long as it's imported It will have distinct seasons of growth.

The cloves are planted in the time of harvest (fall). The greens and roots develop during winter. At this point, in the warmer conditions, bulbs begin to thicken out. As the greens are shrinking, harvest them and tuck the wilted greens and hang them on a pillar of the carport.

The process of planting is easy. Sort out all the cloves within each bulb. In the event that your garden has a bed that is around 2 feet. length it is possible to plant in lines. Instead, plant in symmetrical triangular shapes of 4 inches sides. For a different way of thinking you can plant the circles in concentric circles that are less than 4 inches in distance and each clove is approximately four crawls away from neighbors along the lines. The result is, all likelihood, is a separation. To set them in the ground, drive the piece that is level at the bottom into the ground, and the sharp piece on top just running across the dirt.

Take care of your property is important, but try to keep it from becoming become dry. Be careful not to let the shade off your harvests.

Take them in before the greens begin to shrivel completely during a hot, dry day. Get rid of the dirt; do not drag them away to the greens. Put them in a drying rack (don't rinse them) Be on the lookout for them to make sure they don't become decayed. Remove any rotten bulbs straight away. Cut off bulbs when you'll need them.

Garlic is a good source of:

* Reduce your strain on your circulatory system.

* Manage your glucose levels

• Remove heavy elements from the body

* Kills molds and microbes.

* Sometimes, even fights infections that Antibiotics aren't able to do.

* Helps fight yeast contamination

* Fights diseases

It is evident that garlic is a mix of many different supplements, however the one that has the greatest health benefits could result the most benefits when you open it up to air.

Put your garlic in an masher, and then expose the mashing to the air for a few minutes before using it. As an example, I've put one pound of garlic in the press to create stew, then let it spread across a large plate as I cook the rest portion of my stew. I usually make two Gallons of stew in one go and then freeze the divided portions.

There's even huge mild garlic that we call Russian garlic. It is possible to cook an apple-sized bulb and consume it as a dish of vegetables. In any way you choose to utilize it, make sure you don't leave out garlic from your preparations to cultivate your vegetable naturally.

People who have Natural tallness often seek ways to get taller. If you are naturally tall then you might be doing the same. When you're looking around, you'll discover a variety of ways to get taller. however, there are certain items you need to be aware of to ensure that you have the most effective results of your attempts to get more taller. What exactly are they? Peruse on and find out.

Do not take any medication or Antibiotics which hinder in the release of the hormone that helps human development. If the production of the development hormone is reduced and your growth will be halted and you will not be able grow more taller. Also, it is recommended not take any medication and medical procedures that can help you increase your height. They can cause a number of negative signs for your physique.

Do not take any fake development hormones. It will trigger a myriad of reactions that can affect your overall health. The most common methods are the efficient methods for increasing the production of hormones. Different methods can be dangerous therefore, avoid them.

Be sure to supplement your diet with nutrients and calcium supplements during the development phase. It is essential to provide the required amounts of calcium to your body to improve the health of your bones. This isn't likely to be achievable in your daily food intake, so be sure you're also taking regular calcium supplements. There are many other enhancements that can allow you to provide all vital nutrients your body needs start utilizing these.

Averting from an eating plan which is packed with protein and calcium is possibly the most dangerous mix-up that you could get into. The mere act of doing nothing will not have the ability to help you in becoming more taller. You must adhere to an appropriate diet in order to reap the maximum benefits from your activities. It is also important to be sure to not cut off your right to sleep.

Avoid slouching your back. This affects your posture in a way. It's time to get into the habit of maintaining your spine in a straight line. This also provides a good stretching of your back. If you are prone to an off-base posture it is difficult to achieve this initially. However it will get you acclimated to it slowly. A good posture can be achieved by maintaining your spine straight. Keep your your stomach in, and your jawline raised.

If you've looked through the above mentioned botches then you have a better likelihood of growing more taller. In addition, it's crucial to think about being taller, and you'll believe that it is easier to implement the methods to increase your height and stay focussed on them.

Chapter 15: Natural Cleaner For Everyday Use

Cleaning supplies are among the most important places where the Keepers of the Home want to get rid of toxic chemicals and synthetic compounds that are a part of our household units.

Making my own hand-crafted routine cleaning solutions was a smart first stepsince I am a fan of to plan my work this is what is required to make your own chemical!

I spent hours looking on the web for ideas, plans as well as plans, and tips on handmade cleaners. After many hours of experimentation I've come across very few that I use regularly I'm sharing these today to ensure that you won't have to complete all the legwork!

Before we get into the specific strategies I'll just say that White vinegar as well as heating drinks can clean almost everything! It's the main ingredient in many of the plans below but there are a myriad of objects that it could clean and more!

In this way, therefore it is time to begin with the kitchen.

Most-used cleaner is a effective cleaner that is fantastic for a broad range of surfaces that are hard:

Custom-designed All-Purpose Cleaner

* 1/2 cup white vinegar

* 2 Tbsp heating pop

* 10 drops lavender, tea tree or lemon essential oil

Directions:

Blend the vinegar, the basic oils, and a bit of water prior to making soft drinks . Do this in a sparkling bathtub (glass is the best choice).

Then you can fill the bottle to the top with water. I typically use 12 oz bottles.

Shake gently to mix recipes. Then splash, then wipe with the material, and allow drying.

Custom-designed "Delicate Scrub" Cleaner

* 1/2 cup of ingredients for making pop

* 1 cup ecologically-resistant fluid cleansing cleanser for clothing

* 10 drops lavender, tea tree or lemon essential oil

Directions:

Blend prepared pop and cleanser for clothes in a bowl of blending and mix vigorously to combine to create glue. Add oil base and mix well. Store in a air-tight water or food container.

* In the event that the mix begins to dry, add only a tiny amount of water and mix well.

Custom made Disinfectant Wipes

*1 cup of water

* 1/4 cup vinegar

* 8 drops of tea tree oil

* 8 drops of eucalyptus fundamental oil

* 8 drops lemon essential oil

* Clean "wipe" container (child wipes, as an example.)

* 15 to 20 squares (old shirt sleeves work well and so do dishtowels from the past or similar material)

Directions:

Spread each square of material in the wipe compartment that is empty and place it in an immune place.

Blend in a bowl vinegar, water and the 3 essential oils, and mix until are well-mixed.

This blend should be poured over the contents of the compartment , where they will absorb and will be ready for you to pull out and utilize!

www.ingramcontent.com/pod-product-compliance
Lightning Source LLC
LaVergne TN
LVHW010936260125
802193LV00009B/853
9781998901500